THIS REMARKABLE B( professionals who are often at a loss when treating patients who are suffering with symptoms that have no organic source. Drs. Abbass and Schubiner have written a clear, concise, and comprehensive text that provides information on the understanding, assessment and treatment of a myriad of mind-body syndromes. It is timely and essential.

—*Patricia Coughlin Ph.D., Author of*
Maximizing Effectiveness in Dynamic Psychotherapy

IN THIS HIGHLY ACCESSIBLE MANUAL of techniques for diagnosing and treating one of the healer's greatest challenges —patients with medically unexplained symptoms—the authors, with the combined wisdom of more than 60 years of practice and teaching, have laid out an invaluable roadmap for developing meaningful, effective and mutually satisfying relationships with patients. A must read for anyone working with patients who present with medically unexplained symptoms.

—*Richard M. Frankel Ph.D., Professor of Medicine and*
*Geriatrics, Indiana University School of Medicine*

HIDDEN FROM VIEW SHARES the clinical wisdom of two of the world's leading scholars on the treatment of chronic pain and other psychophysiological disorders. Drs. Abbass and Schubiner thoroughly describe various techniques for determining whether or not a patient has a psychophysiological disorder. They then present, with clarity yet sophistication, a comprehensive sequence of educational, behavioral, cognitive, and emotional interventions to treat these often challenging and frustrating patients. Physicians and other professionals will find a wealth of useful techniques to incorporate into their practices.

—*Mark A. Lumley, Ph.D., Distinguished Professor and*
*Director of Clinical Psychology Training*
*Department of Psychology, Wayne State University*

*HIDDEN FROM VIEW* contains a wealth of practical experience, medical wisdom and theoretical explanation. It is a must read for all medical professionals in search of more refined ways to listen, observe, evaluate and treat patients with psychophysiologic disorders.

—*Arno L. Goudsmit, Ph.D., School of Family Medicine,*
*Maastricht University, Netherlands*

PSYCHOPHYSIOLOGIC disorders touch every medical specialty so anyone who provides care to patients should read this book. In the emergency department, this is a group of patients whom we have consistently failed. This spectrum of conditions provides a large fraction of the suffering of our patients and should no longer be considered a 'diagnosis of exclusion.' This great book challenges us to recognize features of these disorders and to offer help to patients who have been left to suffer for far too long.

—*Samuel Campbell, MD, Professor of Emergency Medicine*
*Dalhousie University, Canada*

*HIDDEN FROM VIEW* is a book that the field badly needs. Written by two of the leaders in the field, both master clinicians with years of experience with this population, this book contains a wealth of practical and theoretical information that will prove invaluable to any clinician working with somatoform patients, especially primary care physicians and psychotherapists. Particularly notable is the wide variety of creative and effective interventions designed specifically for primary care physicians and other specialists, as well as extensive clinical examples and transcripts of actual psychotherapy sessions with Dr. Abbass. One's understanding of and work with these patients will be significantly enhanced digesting the contents of this outstanding volume.

—*William H. Watson, Ph.D., Associate Professor of Psychiatry*
*(Psychology) and Neurology, University of Rochester*

*HIDDEN FROM VIEW* is a book that every doctor should read. The book includes a complete overview of educational, cognitive, behavioural, and emotional components to help patients see how stress can affect their lives and how biography can have an impact on biology. *Hidden from View* is a book that will change and improve your way to work, helping you achieve successful outcomes with your patients.

—*Erica Poli, MD, EFP Group Integrative Medicine Center,*
*Milan, Italy*

*HIDDEN FROM VIEW* is a must for all clinicians who treat patients with physical symptoms that cannot be explained through a traditional medical model. It is a clear and concise guide that will help you understand, assess and offer brief treatments for the emotional causes underlying what are often seen as medically unexplainable disorders. With this guide, you can begin to feel empowered in your approach to these often-confusing presentations and in so doing, you can begin to empower your patients to address what is truly driving their suffering. This book has the potential to change how you think and how you practice indefinitely.

—*Angela Cooper, Ph.D., Assistant Professor*
*Dalhousie University, Canada*

THIS LANDMARK CONTRIBUTION changes the landscape for how clinicians conceptualize physical health and the connection between emotions and health. A perfect combination of practical and theoretical knowledge, with compelling evidence skillfully woven throughout. *Hidden from View* contains a seemingly radical yet simple approach that should be required reading for all clinicians.

—*E. Adriana Wilson, MD, FRCPC*
*Founder of the Association for Positive Psychiatry of Canada*

PSYCHOPHYSIOLOGIC DISORDERS are common, often unrecognized, and pose major challenges to the primary care physician worried about "missing something." Drs. Abbass and Schubiner in *Hidden From View* offer a practical and direct way to approach these disorders in clinical practice. Chapters on understanding the physiology, evaluating and educating the patient, and providing intervention strategies, both cognitive behavioral and emotion focused, based on Intensive Short-Term Dynamic Psychotherapy, are backed by many examples modeling and explaining their interventions. This book, backed by years of research, will increase the clinician's confidence in approaching and treating these disorders.

*—Bernie Vaccaro, MD, FAPM, Assistant Professor of Psychiatry, Harvard Medical School*

HEALTH PROFESSIONALS frequently encounter painful conditions which do not respond to medical treatment. Yet, until now, they had few tools for helping these patients. This book gives them the tools they need to assess and treat pain conditions which do not respond to traditional medical treatments. Through clinical examples, the authors show how to engage the patient in treatment, how to address resistance, how to help patients face the emotions they usually avoid, and how to regulate anxiety that causes many of these symptoms. Professionals treating chronic pain patients should consider this book a "must read."

*—Jon Frederickson, MSW, Washington School of Psychiatry*

PSYCHOPHYSIOLOGICAL DISORDERS ARE a threefold problem, simultaneously accounting for a large fraction of patients' suffering, overall healthcare spening, and healthcare providers' frustration. In this volume, two of the world's leading experts on the diagnosis and treatment of these illnesses will introduce you to diagnostic techniques and therapeutic interventions that have the potential to dramatically improve all three of these areas.

*—Nat Kuhn, MD, Lecturer in Psychiatry, Harvard Medical School*

Printer: Sheridan Books, Inc.
Printed in the United States of America
Design and Art Direction: Eric Keller
Production Design: Arlene Cohn
Editor: Michael Betzold
Proofreader: George Nolte

Set in Bembo, Benton Sans and Sabon

Abbass, Allan and Schubiner, Howard
Hidden From View: A clinician's guide to psychophysiologic disorders

ISBN-13: 978-0-9843367-8-4
ISBN-10: 0-9843367-8-8

# HIDDEN
## *from*
# VIEW

A CLINICIAN'S GUIDE
TO PSYCHOPHYSIOLOGIC
DISORDERS

Allan Abbass, MD
Howard Schubiner, MD

PSYCHOPHYSIOLOGIC PRESS

To John E. Sarno, MD, a pioneer in the field
of mind body medicine (1923-2017)

# Acknowledgements

ALLAN WOULD LIKE TO acknowledge with gratitude the support of colleagues at the Centre for Emotions and Health, Family Medicine, Emergency Medicine, and Internal Medicine at Dalhousie University, Richard Zehr, Angela Cooper, Joel Town, and Ryan Wilson. Howard acknowledges Mark Lumley at Wayne State University and Alan Gordon at the Pain Psychology Center in Los Angeles as collaborators in research, clinical work and education, and as friends.

We also wish to thank our families; Howard's wife, Val Overholt, for her wise counsel and support and Allan's wife, Jennifer, and children Lauren, Will and Anthony for their steady support.

We want to thank the many colleagues who reviewed drafts of this book and provided feedback. These include Drs. Bianca Horner, Joanna Zed, Angela Cooper, Lothar Matter, Sam Campbell, Arno Goudsmit and colleagues at University of Maastrict Family Medicine, Steven Allder, Patrick Luyten, and Nat Kuhn.

We are very thankful for a talented designer, Eric Keller, an excellent editor, Michael Betzold, and a dedicated proofreader, George Nolte.

We both are deeply indebted to our patients who give us the privilege of knowing them and learning with them on a daily basis how the mind and body function together.

While writing this book we lost a major influence on our work, John E. Sarno, MD. Dr. Sarno was a pioneer in the field of mind body medicine and has made great contributions over the past 40 years. He is greatly missed. His story has recently been documented in the film, All the Rage, by Michael Galinsky. Dr. Sarno has influenced a whole generation of researchers and clinicians to help patients with psychophysiologic disorders. We are proud to be counted among them.

# Table of Contents

HIDDEN FROM VIEW

# Foreword

THIS MANUAL IS BASED ON many years of clinical practice, research, and teaching about diagnosing and managing patients who present with a variety of medically unexplained symptoms which are often due to psychophysiologic disorders (PPD). Psychophysiologic disorders vary from common syndromes such as headache, abdominal discomfort, and back pain to unusual subjective symptoms such as paresthesias, excessive sensitivity to sound, muscle twitching, and unexplained muscle weakness. Unfortunately, in modern medical practice few patients are diagnosed with a PPD; they are hidden from view. However, when you know what to look for, these disorders are obvious.

Our goals are to help you understand the role of emotional processes in your patient's health, learn how to evaluate patients, acquire specific brief office interventions, and recognize when a different level of care or referral is warranted. First, we review essential information concerning the clinical assessment of patients suspected of having psychophysiologic disorders. Then we describe educational and behavioral approaches to counselling patients with PPD. Following that, we discuss the physiology of emotions and illustrate ways emotions can be recognized and evaluated in a clinical interview to improve your assessment, education, and treatment of patients. Finally, we offer brief emotion-focused therapeutic approaches for clinicians. In the final chapter we offer an algorithm explaining when to move to a different step or to refer for more advanced care. While this book comes from the combined experience and efforts of the authors, chapters 2-4 are primarily written by Dr. Schubiner, chapters 5-8 by Dr. Abbass, while both wrote chapters 1 and 9.

This guide is intended to improve your ability to detect and manage emotional, cognitive, and behavioral contributors to illness in the office setting, improving your relationships with patients and your approach to caring for them. This knowledge can reduce excessive medical service use, bolster your confidence as a clinician and improve patient outcomes. In addition, it may improve your own quality of life by helping you reflect on your own emotional and physical well-being.

A wide range of clinicians interact with patients with PPDs. Physicians, physical therapists, occupational therapists, nurse specialists, psychologists, social workers, and other practitioners encounter them daily. We hope that this manual will be useful to all health care providers.

We welcome any feedback about this book.

Allan Abbass, MD and Howard Schubiner, MD
February, 2018

CHAPTER 1

# Overview of Psychophysiologic Disorders

ELIZABETH, A 32-YEAR-OLD WOMAN, *is in your office complaining of episodic shortness of breath, multiple pain symptoms, and transient choking sensations. Two previous workups have not identified a medical disorder. As I interview her about her symptoms, a tear rolls down her cheek.*

PETER, A 45-YEAR-OLD MAN, *has a history of constant low back pain for the past six months. It began several years ago as intermittent pain. It does not radiate to the legs, although he reports an occasional tingling in his anterior thighs. The neurological exam is normal. His MRI shows evidence of degenerative disc disease at three lumbar levels and a bulging disc at L4-5, with moderate neural foraminal narrowing on the left. He has had two courses of physical therapy with little improvement.*

THESE TWO PATIENTS represent commonly encountered presentations that may be due to a psychophysiologic etiology, a structural cause, or a combination of the two. We will use these patients to illustrate how to diagnose and treat these possibilities.

### Overview

Psychological and emotional factors play a role in a significant proportion of family practice visits as well as many specialty consultations (Kroenke, 2003; Kroenke and Rosmalen, 2006; Stuart and Noyes, 1999). A meta-analysis of studies conducted in primary care offices found that between 40% and 49% of patients had at least one medically unexplained symptom and a somatoform disorder could be diagnosed in 26-34% (Haller, et. al., 2015). In fact, psychological and social factors can be the root cause of a wide array of symptoms, including neck and back pain, abdominal and pelvic pain syndromes, fibromyalgia, anxiety, depression, fatigue, insomnia, and autonomic dysfunction syndromes such as irritable bowel or bladder syndrome (Schubiner and Betzold, 2016). Psychosocial factors often play a large role in treatment failures, non-compliance, delayed recovery from injury, and excess use of medical services. Unfortunately, these factors are not often identified nor effectively treated (Kroenke, 2003; Kroenke and Rosmalen, 2006).

In addition to this, emotional factors in the health of providers impact their quality of life and enjoyment of healthcare practice. Patients with treatment-resistant syndromes and significant emotional issues can diminish healthcare provider satisfaction. When this occurs on a regular basis, burnout and medical errors can occur (Croskerry, et. al., 2010).

### Spectrum of Causative Factors

Each patient with psychophysiologic disorders, or PPD, presents with a unique combination of symptoms, histories of adverse life events, reactions to their symptoms, and current life situations. Because of this, PPD can be caused by anything from more easily accessible behavioral, cognitive, and interpersonal factors to more deeply rooted unconscious emotional factors (Table 1.1).

### Learned Phenomena

Some patients with less severe cases of PPD have learned certain patterns of thought and behavior. They worry about their symptoms and behave in other ways that worsen those symptoms. This anxiety often affects voluntary muscles and they often present with tension headaches or neck pain. Their symptoms may be reinforced by others, including health professionals.

These patients may be able to identify emotions generated by past traumas. They are capable of forming healthy attachment relationships. Given insight into how stress and mental processes produce their symptoms, they can usually identify underlying psychological issues and respond to educational, cognitive, and behavioral interventions. Treatment includes a careful explanation of the underlying role of stress and introduction of methods that can alter dysfunctional thoughts and behaviors that contribute to the symptoms. Other approaches may include training in skills needed to recognize and manage stress. These are found in chapters 2-4.

### Unconscious Conflicts

On the more severe end of PPD are those patients whose symptoms are driven primarily by unconscious and emotional processes. These patients often have alexithymia, a primary

### Table 1.1: Spectrum of PPD Causes and Treatments

| Conscious | Unconscious |
|---|---|
| Learned cognitive, behavioral and interpersonal factors | Emotional conflicts, psychic deficits, and poor insight |
| **Healthy Attachments** | **Impaired Attachments** |
| Low trauma load | High trauma load |
| Good anxiety tolerance | Variable-low anxiety tolerance |
| Good emotion access | Poor emotion access: alexithymia |
| Receptive to treatment | Resistant to treatment |
| **Treatments:** | **Treatments:** |
| Educational, cognitive, behavioral, skill building | Emotionally focused Psychodynamic |

difficulty in identifying, experiencing, and expressing emotions. They tend to have a greater symptom load, including anxiety and depression, and a much larger burden of traumatic life events. They may have less insight into the role that emotions play in their symptoms. These patients often fail to respond to traditional medical and psychotherapeutic interventions.

Such patients more likely require therapy that first builds capacities to recognize feelings and understand the links between feelings and symptoms. Such work is described with case studies in chapters 5-8.

## A Continuum

Between these two poles are many patients who will respond to combinations of these two approaches. The more easily learned techniques outlined in chapters 2-4 work well with a majority of primary care patients. Some of these treatment strategies are familiar to many health care providers, particularly those with counseling backgrounds.

Some patients with deeply rooted emotional conflicts can benefit from some of these cognitive, behavioral and educational techniques. Some on the less severe end of the spectrum can also benefit from the emotion-focused therapy described in chapters 5-8. All patients with PPDs will benefit from rational medical workups to rule out structural disorders and clear explanations of how the brain constructs sensations that are experienced.

## Practice Types and Interventions

Many types of clinicians see patients with PPDs. Some work in very busy settings within significant time constraints that limit their time to interview patients. These clinicians will benefit from understanding the many sources of PPD, how to evaluate them, how to deliver some brief education, cognitive, and behavioral interventions and how to recognize when to refer patients for specialized treatment.

Other clinicians who have more time with patients may benefit from learning how to identify underlying causes of PPD, how to deliver cognitive, behavioral, and educational treatments, how to perform detailed psychological diagnoses, and how to help patients recognize and process unconscious feelings.

The interventions we describe in this book cover a range of treatment options and therapies needed to help patients recover from psychophysiologic disorders. It's our hope that each reader will find information useful for their patient population and consistent with their own experiences, interests, and training. However, many health care professionals work in silos and naturally tend to restrict their practice to a limited purview. We have found that to help patients with PPD, many practitioners need to expand their purview; psychotherapists need to understand the biology and neuroscience of PPD while physicians and other healthcare professionals need to understand the psychology of PPD.

## Central Role of a Trusting Relationship

As a foundation for this clinical work, creating trust with your patient is always key. Patients with these disorders are often stigmatized and marginalized by healthcare staff, their symptoms viewed as being "not real" or "all in their heads." Their calls for help can be misconstrued as "pain behaviors" or "secondary gain," and their life circumstances and large symptom load can seem overwhelming. Many psychophysiologic symptoms begin with ruptured attachments in life, that is, adverse early life experiences. When health care providers understand that their pain is real and that the reasons for their symptoms are often rooted in childhood neglect, abandonment, or abuse, it is easier to demonstrate a caring attitude and pay a great deal of attention to developing trust. When examining the following interventions, consider that such a therapeutic relationship with your patient is a necessary ingredient for success at each step. We hope that this book will help you better understand your patients and transmit these concepts as a means of establishing this trust.

## CHAPTER 1 SUMMARY

- *The causes of PPD span a spectrum from learned patterns to deeply rooted emotional processes.*

- *Emotional factors play a role in a significant proportion of patients seen in medical settings. Treatments should be tailored to these causes on an individual basis.*

- *Most health care professionals can benefit from the theory and techniques in this book.*

- *A caring, trusting relationship is critical in managing patients with PPD.*

p. 2 list q Sx & dx.

CHAPTER 2

# Medical Evaluation of the Patient with a Psychophysiologic Disorder

ELIZABETH ARRIVES *for a second visit with a range of symptoms, including headache, neck pain, arm and leg pain, and intermittent diarrhea. Since her last visit, she was seen in the emergency department with shortness of breath. She is distressed and disappointed that she has received no clear answer or help other than pain medications. A CT scan and MRI of the brain are normal; an MRI of her neck shows only minimal degenerative changes; an esophagogastroduodenoscopy (EGD), colonoscopy and serologic tests for celiac disease show no abnormalities. Pulmonary function tests, a CT scan of her lungs, and echocardiogram are also normal. Testing for Lyme disease and for systemic lupus erythematosus and other rheumatologic disorders are normal.*

PETER RETURNS *after seeing a physical medicine and rehabilitation physician. Six weeks of physical therapy helped only minimally. He then had a series of three epidural injections. The first one reduced his pain by 50 percent for one week, but the other injections did not help, and his pain is now back to where it was before the injections. He has consulted two neurosurgeons. One told him that his back was badly damaged, possibly due to genetic factors, and that there was nothing he could do. The other said he could perform surgery if the pain became unbearable. Peter says the pain is getting worse, and he has curtailed almost all physical activities. He is now taking narcotics for pain.*

IN ASSESSING ALL patients, it is critical to distinguish between structural disorders that cause emotional reactions and psychophysiologic disorders caused by stressful life events and emotional responses. While structural physical disorders can cause strong emotional reactions, they are not caused by psychophysiological factors. Many patients have elements of both a structural disease process and a psychophysiologic disorder, but most physicians and other biomedical clinicians ascribe physical illnesses to purely structural processes and do not identify disorders that are primarily or purely psychophysiologic. PPD is common and in many cases can be managed by a primary care physician or other medical or mental health clinicians.

### Common Problems, Common Presentations

Primary healthcare providers commonly encounter pain, fatigue, and other non-specific complaints in the absence of disease or injury (Abbass, et. al., 2009; Rief and Barsky, 2005). An estimated one-third to one-half of outpatient primary care visits are for medically unexplained symptoms (MUS), also termed "functional" disorders, or somatoform disorders (Kroenke, 2003; Kroenke and Rosmalen, 2006; Haller, et. al., 2015; Stuart and Noyes, 1999). These presentations—including a large proportion of patients with headaches, irritable bowel and bladder syndromes, fibromyalgia, chronic fatigue syndrome, and neck and back pain—often overlap and are associated with anxiety, depression, and post-traumatic stress disorder (PTSD) (Amir, et. al., 1997; Beckham, et. al., 1997; Sherman, et. al., 2000). These disorders share aspects of psychiatric comorbidity, functional impairment, and difficult family histories (Aaron and Buchwald, 2001; Henningsen, et. al., 2003). Patients with MUS have significant distress and impairment (Stuart and Noyes, 1999) and are responsible for a major portion of disability in the workforce (Barsky, et. al., 2005; Wessely, et. al., 1999); it is estimated that these disorders cost $100 billion annually in health care in the U.S. (Barsky, et. al., 2005). However, the total costs associated with chronic pain in the U.S. is estimated at $600 billion, more than the costs of cardiac disease, diabetes mellitus and cancer combined (Institute of Medicine, 2011).

There are numerous studies which suggest that early adverse life experiences— including sexual abuse, physical abuse, emotional abuse, and neglect—contribute to the development of psychophysiological disorders in adulthood (Felliti, et. al., 1998; Stuart and Noyes, 1999; Sansone, et. al., 2001; Spertus, et. al., 2003, Sachs-Ericsson, et. al., 2017). Adverse childhood events are associated with chronic pain (Green, et. al., 2001; Goldberg, et. al., 1999), headaches (Raphael, et. al., 2004), gynecological complaints (Cunningham, et. al., 1988), gastrointestinal symptoms (Bass, et. al., 1999), and musculoskeletal symptoms (Bendixen, et. al., 1994).

There is also a strong relationship between medically unexplained symptoms and psychiatric disorders. Significantly higher rates of psychiatric symptoms and diagnoses are found in individuals with fibromyalgia (Aaron, et. al., 1996; Merskey, 1989), irritable bowel syndrome (Thompson, et. al., 1999; Whitehead, et. al., 1988), multiple chemical sensitivities (Barsky and Borus, 1999), and chronic fatigue syndrome (Manu, et. al., 1989; Morrison, 1980). Patients with PPDs have increased rates of depression and anxiety (Bass, et. al., 2001; Katon, et. al., 2001), and somatic symptoms are also significantly increased in patients with depression and anxiety (Kroenke, 2003; Sha, et. al., 2005).

Our premise is that medically unexplained illnesses are psychophysiologic: the brain creates these symptoms in response to psychological stress via *learned neural pathways*. The physical symptoms are not caused by structural disorders or pathological processes but rather by reversible physiological processes. The determination of PPD can be made only after organic factors are ruled out through a detailed history and physical examination as well as judicious use and careful interpretation of laboratory and imaging procedures.

## The Neurophysiology of PPD

The brain can cause a wide array of mild to severe symptoms in virtually any area of the body. The central mechanisms of psychophysiologic disorders have become better understood in recent years. Timothy Noakes, an exercise physiologist, has studied how the brain reacts to running a marathon (Noakes, 2001). Dr. Noakes explained why well-trained athletes "hit the wall" in endurance events: when they get pain and fatigue during a race, their brain is sounding an alarm warning them that they will run out of energy soon by recruiting fewer muscles for activity by neural pathways. Noakes calls this the central governor function of the brain and explains that athletes must ignore these warning signals in order to finish the race, recognizing that there is no actual danger of physical harm. "Hitting the wall" is like when the light on your car's dashboard goes on to warn you that your gas is getting low; your car can still run fine for quite a while.

*"This new understanding of fatigue brings together all the different models of exercise physiology. In fact, the findings of the separate models can all be explained by the action of a central governor that regulates exercise to ensure that internal body homeostasis is maintained and bodily damage avoided. Fatigue is merely the emotional expression of the subjective symptoms that develop as these subconscious controls wage a fierce battle with the conscious mind to ensure that the conscious ultimately submits to the superior will of the subconscious (Noakes, 2001)."*

Gracely and Schweinhardt (2015) offer another way of understanding the role of the brain in producing pain, fatigue, and other psychophysiologic symptoms by using the concept of promoted quiescence (PQ).

As the human brain developed, predators were the main threats to our well-being. If a lion begins to chase you, you have a powerful "fight or flight" reaction. This highly activated state allows us to use all available resources, including muscle activation and mental focus, to protect ourselves. You can't sustain this state long, but during these episodes individuals generally feel no pain or fatigue even if injured. Afterwards, the brain activates a state of rest and recovery, *creating* fatigue, pain, and cognitive dysfunction to enforce inactivity. This important adaptive state typically lasts for a few days to a few weeks, depending on the degree of injury. As the injuries heal, the brain "turns off" the danger signal of pain and fatigue to allow a return to full activity.

In the modern world, the threats and dangers are often ongoing emotional and stressful situations. Since the brain responds to emotional injury in the same manner as physical injury (Kross, et. al., 2011; Eisenberger, et. al., 2006), when one experiences significant stressful life events, the brain may activate the rest- and recovery-response for a prolonged time. In the state of promoted quiescence, the brain warns us of an ongoing danger by continuing to create symptoms such as pain, fatigue, and impaired cognition. It is very easy to misinterpret these reactions as being due to ongoing structural damage. This is the prevailing view of patients and health care providers, even if the injury has healed and significant time has passed.

Research by Apkarian and colleagues has solidified the link between emotions and chronic pain. Enhanced connectivity in an emotionally laden neural pathway between the nucleus accumbens and the prefrontal cortex, as seen on fMRIs, was predictive of chronic back pain in those with a subacute back injury (Baliki, et. al., 2012). It is likely that these pathways represent learned neural pathways caused by prior traumatic life events. In addition, those with chronic back pain have fMRI evidence of activation of emotional areas rather than somatosensory (nociceptive) areas (Hashmi, et. al., 2013).

The subconscious brain is the driving force behind psychophysiologic reactions. The subconscious controls our bodily functions to protect us, to ward off unacceptable feelings and help us adapt to our environment. Our reactions to our environment depend on both the innate and learned coding of our brain. Over our lifetime, our brain learns to respond to potentially dangerous situations. And, as Hebb famously noted, "when neurons fire together, they become wired together," and those neural pathways become more likely to fire the more they are activated (Hebb, 1949).

Our brain controls not only responses to our environment but also what we perceive. Eyewitness accounts are dramatically altered by the values and experiences of the viewer (Arkowitz and Lilienfeld, 2010; Drew, et. al., 2013; Lum, et. al., 2005; Morgan, et. al., 2004). We can see only what our brains expect us to see. This is known as predictive coding: what we perceive is predicted from past experiences. For visual, auditory and taste perceptions, this is termed exteroception. A similar process, interoception, occurs for internal sensations (Feldman Barrett and Simmons, 2015): the brain creates the sensations it expects us to feel. When the brain is in an ongoing state of warning, danger, and promoted quiescence, it will continue to produce pain with movement, fatigue with activity, disordered thought processes, and many other sensations designed to enforce rest and inactivity. And the more the accompanying neural pathways are activated, the more they become normalized as default pathways. The brain can continue to produce psychophysiologic symptoms long after the threat of danger has dissipated. Pain and other symptoms are messages that we receive from our subconscious brain. Pain can occur in the absence of physical injury (Fisher, et.al., 1995), and not all physical injuries result in pain (Beecher, 1951). In some cases, pain represents actual tissue damage, while in others it is a signal of perceived danger that has a complex neurological and psychological causation. For more information on predictive coding, interoception, and how the brain constructs what we feel, see Feldman Barrett (2017).

## Preparing the Way

Your efforts to examine links between stress and illness can be met with resistance from many patients but you can do a few things to reduce this resistance. First, develop trust through listening with a caring and sympathetic attitude towards patients (Fonagy and Allison, 2014). Such a trusting relationship is therapeutic and critically important when evaluating patients with PPDs. Second, prepare patients for inevitable conversations about stress and health through adding questions to new patient intake forms such as "Have you encountered a great deal of stress in your life?," "How much stress are you experiencing at this time?," "Have you noticed that your symptoms are worse when you are more stressed?," and "Where do you tend to hold stress in your body?" Just as a family history is typically included in intake forms, a modified Holmes and Rahe scale (Holmes and Rahe, 1967) can help if it covers a lifelong history of stressful and traumatic events. Another useful screening questionnaire is The Patient Health Questionnaire Somatic, Anxiety, and Depressive Symptom Scale (PHQ-SADS) (Kroenke, et. al., 2010). Third, pamphlets about the physical impact of stress can be kept in your waiting area. With these signals up front, patients will not be surprised during the office visit when you ask about stress as a contributor to somatic symptoms. Finally, tell patients that emotional stress affects the body so they realize this is a normal process that you will consider: explain to them you are examining how their body responds to stress. This conversation will help allay anxiety that you are accusing them of making up symptoms or imagining symptoms. These steps can make an emotion-based assessment palatable for patients.

### Initial Clinical Considerations

Be aware of the potential for PPD in all patients and be prepared to closely examine the patient's history to determine if symptoms are reflective of an organic disease (a pathological process), a psychophysiologic process or a combination of the two. Just as you see circulation as a basic physical function, it's important to assess patients' emotional capacities—such as the ability to identify and express emotions and their psychological strengths, such as resilience in the face of adversity.

Do not assume that a painful condition of any duration or severity must be due to a structural process. Psychophysiologic processes can and do cause chronic, severe pain. Sudden chest pain can certainly be caused by angina or a myocardial infarction, but it may also be a reaction to a stressful life event that creates unconscious anxiety that, in turn, activates pain. In the same way, chronic back or head pain can be due to a PPD. In fact, it is likely that PPD is the primary cause of pain when no specific disease process has been identified with a careful history, physical examination, and judicious use of laboratory testing and imaging. It is obviously critical to make the distinction between organic diseases and psychophysiologic disorders; the treatments are vastly different.

Clearly, certain patterns of symptoms are highly suggestive of a pathologic disease, such as sudden onset of severe, colicky flank pain associated with blood in the urine—likely indicating kidney stones. However, there is evidence of a significant role of stress and the power of the mind in disorders usually thought of as purely physical. For example, higher resting activation of the amygdala has been shown to be predictive of cardiac disease (Tawakol, et. al., 2017). A study of patients with moderate to severe Parkinson's disease showed that a placebo injection labelled as an "expensive new medication" had significant objective effects on motor function (Espay, et. al., 2015). In other studies, the mindset of participants was shown to alter physiologic effects of exercise (changes in blood pressures and body mass index) and metabolism of food (changes in ghrelin levels) (Crum and Langer, 2007; Crum, et. al., 2011).

ELIZABETH DESCRIBES *left temple headaches and choking sensations that are intermittent. She also has dull, aching pains in her neck, arms, and legs that seem to alternate from one location to another on a frequent basis. There are no clear exacerbating and relieving factors; however, the pains are much worse after exercise. There is no shortness of breath on exertion. Upon further questioning, she notes that she began to have headaches and a "nervous stomach" as a child.*

PETER NOTES THAT *the back pain is better in the morning when he wakes up but gets worse during the day. He avoids any unnecessary movements. Over the past two weeks, the pain has spread into the lower part of the thorax, primarily in the paraspinal areas bilaterally. An MRI of the thoracic spine was normal. The only time he noted a large difference in his pain was when he was on a boat with some of his male friends. During that time, he recalled that he had no back pain for a couple of hours.*

The first and foremost job of a medical evaluation is to identify pathological conditions. Careful histories and physical exams, along with the use of targeted testing, will usually determine if there is a significant structural abnormality. Once a clear pathological process is ruled out, it becomes highly likely that the patient has a psychophysiologic disorder. While ruling out a pathologic process is critical, it is equally important to *rule in* a psychophysiologic process; this process will be reviewed in chapters 5 and 6. Certain conditions are much more likely to be caused by psychophysiologic processes; a partial listing of these disorders is in table 2.1. Patients should be made aware that the brain can cause muscle tension, contractions of bowel or bladder, rapid heart rate, and many other physical processes; and that the brain controls these functions constantly.

### History Taking

Take a careful history looking for clues that point either to a structural problem or a psychophysiologic disorder. The initial onset of a PPD often occurs upon waking from sleep or without any obvious injury. Pain syndromes that do not correspond to known conditions are common in PPD. For example, pain, tingling, or numbness affecting all five fingers of the hand bilaterally is unlikely to be caused by a specific nerve root lesion. Pain that extends down one whole side of the torso or body, pain that radiates from the back of the head to the face, and pain that radiates from the lower back up the spine to the neck are not likely to be structural in nature. Pain that begins in one area and then spreads over time to adjacent areas is likely caused by PPD. It is particularly common for pain or other symptoms of PPD to be bilateral in distribution, often starting on one side before spreading to the other side.

On occasion, psychophysiologic symptoms are spread by social contagion. Research shows that social contagion can contribute to smoking, obesity, and mood disorders (Christakis and Fowler, 2013). A study found that the rates of back pain were much lower in East Germany than in West Germany in the years immediately after the two countries were reunited in 1989. But twenty years later, the rates of back pain were similar in both parts of Germany (Raspe, et. al., 2008).

## Table 2.1: Syndromes Commonly Due to Psychophysiologic Processes

**Chronic Pain Syndromes**
Tension headaches
Migraine headaches
Back pain
Neck pain
Whiplash
Fibromyalgia
Temporomandibular joint (TMJ) syndrome
Chronic abdominal and pelvic pain syndromes
Chronic tendonitis
Vulvodynia
Piriformis syndrome
Sciatic pain syndrome
Repetitive strain injury
Foot pain syndromes
Myofascial pain syndrome

**Autonomic Nervous Symptom Disorders**
Irritable bowel syndrome
Interstitial cystitis (Irritable bladder syndrome)
Postural orthostatic tachycardia syndrome (POTS)
Inappropriate sinus tachycardia
Reflex sympathetic dystrophy (Complex regional pain syndrome)

**Other Syndromes**
Insomnia
Chronic fatigue syndrome, systemic exertion intolerance disease*
Paresthesias (numbness, tingling, burning)
Tinnitus
Dizziness
Spasmodic dysphonia
Chronic hives
Anxiety
Depression
Obsessive-compulsive disorder
Post-traumatic stress disorder
Eating disorders
Substance use disorders
Hypersensitivity syndromes (to touch, sound, smells, foods, medications)

NOTE: *Most of the above disorders can also be caused by structural disease processes.*

*\* Systemic exertion intolerance disease has been identified by the Institute of Medicine as an organic disorder. There remains controversy about this disorder and its relation to chronic fatigue syndrome.*

Take note of variation in symptom patterns. Symptoms that shift from one body part to another or come and go at various times during the day or week are likely to be caused by a psychophysiologic process rather than by pathological conditions. Symptoms that are clearly aggravated by stress or emotions are usually due to PPD. For example, symptoms of PPD often occur in conjunction with stressful events, such as visiting family, going to school or work, approaching deadlines, or having (or anticipating) difficult conversations. Psychophysiologic symptoms often begin or worsen when beginning a trip (particularly when anticipating stress on a car or plane ride or visiting friends or relatives) or returning from a vacation to a stressful family or work situation. Exciting and positive life events, such as having a baby or getting a promotion, can also activate PPD. Symptoms of PPD often have physical triggers, such as having pain when sitting in certain chairs but not others, or during certain activities that are physically demanding but not others. For example, one patient had severe pain while sitting at work but no pain while riding a bicycle.

Chronological patterns can point toward the presence of PPD. For example, a patient with a history of intermittent headaches on workdays but not on weekends—without any signs or symptoms of sinusitis, increased intracranial pressure, fever, or neurological deficits—is likely to have a psychophysiologic disorder (assuming there is no occupational exposure or abnormal lab or imaging results). Another patient who had pain in her hands during the work week while typing noted that the pain also occurred on Sunday evening, even though she had not been typing. Symptoms that disappear when on vacation, on weekends or at random moments are highly likely to be due to PPD. A patient had constant low back pain for several years yet no pain while on a weeklong vacation. Symptoms aggravated by weather changes, specific foods, light, or aromas are likely to be psychophysiologic. Hence, it is critical to probe for times when the symptoms are lessened or absent or shift in location.

PPDs also tend to shift over time: when one set of symptoms lessens, another one begins or is exacerbated. Headaches may abate when abdominal pain begins, or vice versa. One patient had severe abdominal pains several days out of each week. Yet during a six-month period while being treated for breast cancer, she had no episodes. A patient had severe muscle tics that were impairing almost all activities, yet when he played in the orchestra, they were absent.

Patients often ask how the brain "decides" what symptoms to create in response to stressful events. There's often no clear answer. Sometimes symptoms are symbolic. I once saw a woman who had pain in her buttocks. When I asked when it started, she replied, "Right when my husband retired." Foot pain can be symbolic of "needing to put my foot down" and abdominal pain can represent "something that makes me sick."

PPD can be caused by expectations and appear contagious. I know a man who began a graduate program full of fear of getting repetitive strain injury (RSI) from doing a lot of typing. He had read an article about the dangers of RSI, and within a few months developed pain in both wrists. We have seen several patients whose symptoms began after they read an article about the symptom or found out someone they knew had that symptom. Prior injuries are common sites of PPD pain. The brain has "learned" that pain and remembered that pain as a neural pathway that can be easily activated under stress. Many people develop symptoms that occur in other members of their family. This may not be a genetic disorder along the lines of cystic fibrosis or sickle cell anemia, but rather the kind of epigenetic inheritance that is often seen with migraine headaches—a predisposition activated by environmental cues and stress. The brain is modeling certain symptoms that "run in the family." Finally, many PPD symptoms occur in often-used muscles that the brain chooses as places to create chronic pain there, such as the lower back or neck.

Another clue to the diagnosis of PPD is the onset or exacerbation of a physical symptom, such as abdominal cramping or neck pain, while discussing particularly stressful events during the interview. Hence, the somatic effects of emotions can be examined directly in the interview (see chapters 5 and 6).

## Physical Examination and Interpretation of Tests

Some of the most common presenting symptoms are neck and back pain and other musculoskeletal pain syndromes. In these situations, physical examination is critical to check for signs of nerve root compression, such as objective evidence of loss of sensation, change in deep tendon reflexes, or muscle weakness. Point tenderness or limitation in range of motion (of the hip joint, for example) may point to a structural process, especially if diagnostic imaging studies corroborate those findings. However, tight muscles or pain with forward or side bending of the back are common physical findings in people with PPD. Significant pain that occurs with light pressure on tender points, such as seen in fibromyalgia, is highly likely to be due to PPD. Pressure to a specific area that causes pain that radiates to a broader area or an area not connected by typical nerve patterns is characteristic of PPD. For example, in patients with PPD pressure on the trapezius muscle on one side may generate pain that radiates into the top of the head or to the eye on one side or pain that radiates down into the lower back.

Abnormalities on X-ray, CT, or MRI studies are commonly identified in musculoskeletal disorders. But a majority of healthy adults *without* back pain have MRIs that reveal abnormalities such as degenerative discs, bulging and herniated discs, mild degrees of spinal stenosis and spondylolisthesis, scoliosis, Tarlov cysts, and other conditions (Boos, et. al., 2000; Borenstein, et. al., 2001; Brinjikji, et. al., 2015). In one study, 50 percent of healthy 21-year-olds with no pain had evidence of degenerative discs, and 25 percent had a bulging disc (Takatalo, et. al., 2009). Brinjikji and colleagues (see table 2.2) found that 80 percent of 50-year-olds with no history of back pain have evidence of disc degeneration, 60 percent have bulging discs, and 36 percent have herniated discs (Brinjikji, et. al., 2015). Apart from spinal tumors, infections, or fractures, MRI findings in patients with and without back or neck pain are not different. Yet many physicians and physical therapists still commonly assume that the cause of these abnormalities on MRIs is structural. Clearly that is not necessarily true.

## Table 2.2: Occurence of Musculoskeletal Imaging Findings by Age in Asymptomatic Individuals

| Age (yr)            | 20  | 30  | 40  | 50  | 60  | 70  | 80  |
| ------------------- | --- | --- | --- | --- | --- | --- | --- |
| DISK DEGENERATION   | 37% | 52% | 68% | 80% | 88% | 93% | 96% |
| DISK BULGE          | 30% | 40% | 50% | 60% | 69% | 77% | 84% |
| DISK PROTRUSION     | 29% | 31% | 33% | 36% | 38% | 40% | 43% |
| ANNULAR FISSURE     | 19% | 20% | 22% | 23% | 25% | 27% | 29% |
| FACET DEGENERATION  | 4%  | 9%  | 18% | 32% | 50% | 69% | 83% |
| SPONDYLOLISTHESIS   | 3%  | 5%  | 8%  | 14% | 23% | 35% | 50% |

*Printed with permission; The* American Journal of Neuroradiology.

It is important, of course, to recognize clearly pathologic conditions causing back pain, such as tumors, infections, fractures, and referred pain from intra-abdominal or intra-thoracic structures. Equally important is recognizing herniated discs or other abnormalities that cause pressure on the spinal cord (leading to difficulties with bowel or bladder function) or on spinal nerve roots, causing decrease in muscle strength, altered deep tendon reflexes, or loss of sensation. These findings obviously suggest a pathologic process. Nerve root compression is often accompanied by pain and numbness in the affected nerve root distribution. But when the clinical examination reveals no objective signs of nerve root compression and the pain does not correspond to the MRI findings, the pain is likely to be caused by PPD, especially if the history suggests that a PPD can be "ruled in."

About 85 percent of patients with lower back pain do not have a clear pathologic process accounting for their symptoms (Deyo, et. al., 1992). In the modern era, back pain is one of the most common PPD symptoms and has been shown to be more associated with psychological variables than with physical or MRI variables (Carragee, et. al., 2005; Christensen and Knardahl, et. al., 2012). In addition, changes on X-rays due to osteoarthritis are poorly correlated with the degree of joint pain (Creamer and Hochberg, 1998). Therefore, the history and physical examination are crucial in determining if neck, back, or joint pain is likely caused by a structural disorder, a psychophysiologic disorder, or a combination of the two. Osteoarthritis can produce pain, but if the pain is excessive or is inconsistent, PPD may be the culprit, especially if the symptoms and history point to such a diagnosis.

Use a similar process with other symptoms. If a patient has numbness in the arms, legs, hands, and/or feet, but there is no specific nerve root distribution or a systemic disorder causing peripheral neuropathy (such as diabetes mellitus or alcoholism) and there are no objective findings of loss of sensation by pinprick or light touch, a diagnosis of PPD is warranted. Patients with psychophysiologic disorders often present with bilateral and symmetric pain or other symptoms. Sometimes specific pathological conditions can account for such symmetric symptoms, but our experience suggests they are more likely due to brain activation caused by stressful life events. A common scenario is that a patient develops pain in one limb that later occurs in the opposite limb. Widespread joint and muscle pains require investigations for rheumatologic disorders, and head pain requires assessment for intracranial, sinus, or dental disorders. Gastrointestinal and genitourinary symptoms are often due to PPD; routine testing can usually rule out a structural disorder. Medical diagnoses of tension or migraine headaches, fibromyalgia, irritable bowel or bladder syndromes, or pelvic floor dysfunction do not indicate a specific pathological process—they simply describe the symptoms. A careful search for causes of chronic fatigue syndrome or systemic exercise intolerance disease (SEID) is critical. Many patients with chronic fatigue syndrome have recovered using the methods outlined in this manual.

THE PHYSICAL EXAMINATION *on Elizabeth is completely normal except for muscle tenderness in her temples, occiput, neck, arms, and legs. There is no joint swelling, excessive joint laxity, or signs of inflammation. However, she did show signs of hypersensitivity to light touch in several areas. She also described pain radiating bilaterally down her arms with light pressure on one side of the neck.*

PETER'S EXAM REVEALS *normal deep tendon reflexes, normal muscle strength, and normal sensation. He has mild to moderate pain with forward and lateral bending in the lower back. His MRI findings of degenerative changes and a bulging disc are unlikely to explain the pain patterns he displays, since the foraminal narrowing is only on one side and would not affect the nerve roots supplying the anterior thighs. In addition, the pain has spread upwards along his spine and the MRI findings of the thoracic spine were normal. The abnormal MRI findings in his lumbar spine are seen in approximately 50-70% of asymptomatic people of his age.*

### Symptom Checklists

Additional aspects of the history can reveal further evidence pointing to a PPD. Table 2.1 has a checklist of symptoms and disorders commonly caused by PPD. Patients with a history of such disorders, even if now resolved, are much more likely to have PPD.

Here are the results of review of symptoms questionnaires that Elizabeth and Peter completed. (See the appendix for the questionnaire.)

ELIZABETH'S HISTORY SHOWS *headaches, abdominal pain, and anxiety dating back to childhood; neck pain, dizziness, and depression beginning as a teenager; and fibromyalgia, irritable bowel syndrome, pelvic pain, and fatigue beginning in her 20s.*

PETER'S FORM SHOWS *IBS as a teen, anxiety and back pain in his 20s, and frequent urination and tinnitus in his 30s.*

Reviewing these forms, the clinician can often see a pattern that is likely to help explain the current symptoms. In Elizabeth's case, the large number of symptoms that date back to childhood strongly suggests a psychophysiologic origin and the likelihood of significant trauma in her childhood. For Peter, although there are a smaller number of symptoms (he has likely had fewer serious adverse childhood events), the occurrence of back pain with a prior history of IBS, anxiety, and other symptoms also suggests a pattern of PPD. It is unusual to see three or four different structural diseases, especially at early ages, in the absence of a unifying diagnosis, such as multiple sclerosis, cystic fibrosis, systemic lupus erythematosus, sickle cell anemia, HIV/AIDS, or other systemic disorders. When those types of disorders are ruled out and there is a relatively long list of disorders spanning different organ systems, PPD is highly likely. It has been well documented that the disorders in table 2.1, frequently called central sensitization disorders, often occur together (Yunus, 2007; Geisser, et. al., 2008). The parsimony principle (Occam's razor), basic to all science, recommends applying the simplest explanation that fits the evidence. Patients with psychophysiologic disorders have often been given multiple diagnoses to explain their symptoms. But with a wide array of symptoms commonly seen in PPD, the diagnosis is usually quite clear. When patients hear this explanation, they can begin to see that they have fewer things "wrong" with them than they may have been led to believe. Having one syndrome that is potentially reversible is better than having multiple disorders that have not been ameliorated despite extensive medical treatment. You can sort out this confusion for each PPD patient by providing a clear diagnosis with a hopeful prognosis.

### Assessment of Childhood Events

As mentioned, patients with histories of adverse childhood events are much more likely to present with PPD. Studies have shown that individuals with fibromyalgia, migraine headaches, irritable bowel syndrome, interstitial cystitis (painful bladder syndrome), and pelvic pain have high rates of early childhood difficulties (Goodwin, et. al., 2003; Sumanen, et. al., 2007; Latthe, et. al., 2006; Meltzer-Brody, et. al., 2007; Mayer, et. al., 2001). There are strong correlations and overlap between this group of disorders and post-traumatic stress disorder (Dobie, et. al., 2004; Amir, et. al., 1997; Sherman, et. al., 2000; Beckham, et. al., 1997). Sufferers may have histories of emotional, physical, and/or sexual abuse; neglect, abandonment, divorce, parental loss; bullying, significant sibling rivalry or cruelty; illness or death of family members; or other prominent events. These types of trauma can cause the child to have blocked off, anxiety-laden feelings that are later triggered by stressors mentioned above. On a physiological level, these stressors create the emotional pathways of sensitized and exaggerated fight-or-flight/danger/alarm signals easily triggered by later life stress, resulting in PPD. However, many patients have psychophysiologic disorders who do not have significant early life adversity. Everyone has some degree of adversity and even mild forms of difficulties, such as having parents who can be critical or have high expectations, can cause significant resentment and low self-esteem (Assor, et. al., 2004), which creates the foundation for PPD later in life. In addition, some people are much more sensitive to criticism or conditional love than others.

A simple way to begin to identify childhood stressors is to include these three questions on an intake form: 1. Please describe your father (or other male caregivers). 2. Please describe your mother (or other female caregivers). 3. Did you have any traumatic events in childhood?

HERE ARE THE ANSWERS *to these questions from Elizabeth Father—kind, hard working, generous, aloof, strict. Mother— religious, caring, nurturing, worrying, perfectionistic. Traumatic events—Yes—sexual abuse as a child by an adult male who was a neighbor.*

HERE ARE PETER'S ANSWERS:
*Father—hardworking, alcoholic, cruel when drunk, verbally abusive to my mother, good provider, hit me with a belt. Mother—also an alcoholic, but loving, kind, could be critical and judging. No other specific traumatic events in childhood.*

The Adverse Childhood Events (ACE) scale (Fellitti, et. al., 1998) is predictive of a wide variety of disorders in adulthood, such as anxiety, depression, somatic symptoms, and suicide attempts, as well as cardiac disorders, chronic obstructive pulmonary disease, and diabetes mellitus (Anda, et. al., 2006).

See the appendix for the ACE scale, a valid and efficient way to obtain this information.

### Linking Onset Of Psychophysiologic Symptoms With Stressful Life Events

Since PPD symptoms are typically triggered by stress, it's useful to ask if the onset of symptoms occurred at the time of a significant stressful event. Inquire about stressful events at the time of the onset of each of the symptoms found in the review of symptoms checklist, if you have the time for this. It might take a while for the patient to reflect or ask family members for help in recalling what was going on. See the appendix for a description of this "life trajectory" interview. This can be accomplished in smaller chunks of time if necessary.

FOR ELIZABETH, *the onset of childhood symptoms (headaches, abdominal pain, and anxiety) coincided with the onset of the sexual abuse. The symptoms (neck pain, dizziness, and depression) that began in her teens occurred when she was betrayed by a boyfriend who began dating her best girlfriend, ruining both of those relationships. As time passed, she kept the sexual abuse a secret, leading to a great deal of guilt and shame. In her early 20s, she began working at a job where she experienced a great deal of pressure to succeed and felt isolated from co-workers. That's when the fibromyalgia, IBS, and fatigue began. When she started having symptoms of a choking sensation and intermittent difficulty in breathing, she was dating a man who was verbally abusive and once placed his hands around her neck and forced her to have sex with him.*

IN PETER'S CASE, *the IBS symptoms began as a teen, when his parents divorced and he was placed in the middle of their acrimonious battle. In his 20s, he had the onset of back pain and anxiety when he started working for a demanding, critical boss. The recent episode of back pain began when his son began drinking and using drugs, creating conflict in his home and instability in his marriage.*

## Personality Traits

Individuals with PPD usually have similar personality traits. Those with traumatic or emotionally neglectful childhoods are more likely to have low self-esteem. They tend to be self-critical and engage in people-pleasing behaviors. They have high expectations of themselves and put pressure on themselves to succeed, always engage in the "correct" actions, and put other people first. They tend to be very vigilant and take difficulties and criticism very personally. They carry guilt with them and are not assertive about getting their needs met or their opinions heard. These traits further activate the danger and fear pathways of the brain, which can lead to pain and other symptoms. Since these personality patterns begin early in life, many who have them do not recognize them as learned patterns that contribute to the development of PPD. A checklist of these personality traits is included in the appendix.

BOTH ELIZABETH AND PETER *had the majority of these traits, including a strong need to please others, sensitivity to criticism, high expectations for self, perfectionism, a tendency to feel guilty, low self-esteem, and being overly responsible and conscientious.*

## Making the Diagnosis

With patients like Elizabeth and Peter, the absence of a clear pathological disorder, along with childhood adverse effects and the correlation of onset of symptoms with stressful life events, are strong evidence of PPD. However, in some cases, additional focused interviewing may be necessary.

A detailed psychological interview can help both you and the patient understand exactly how and why the PPD symptoms are related to stressful events. This interview can be completed in components over time. You may already have or will develop the skills to conduct these interviews (chapters 5-8). If not, then a referral to a mental health clinician or specialty psychiatric service dedicated to evaluating medically unexplained symptoms may be needed. However, be careful to avoid antagonizing the patient if they do not understand the nature of psychophysiologic processes. It is critical to work closely with the patient and to gain their trust that your only concern is their well-being and recovery. A full description of an approach to this exploration can be found in *Unlearn Your Pain* (Schubiner and Betzold, 2016). This process can help the patient see the connections between emotional patterns, life events, and PPD symptoms.

Most patients are unfamiliar with the concept that the brain can activate powerful physical reactions. After months or years of symptoms that can range from mild to devastating, it is often a big leap to see these symptoms as a psychophysiologic disorder. It is often wise to take some time to let this information sink in and continue to investigate the symptoms to clearly rule out or rule in the appropriate diagnoses.

At times, it's necessary to delay making this diagnosis. Paying close attention to when symptoms are exacerbated and alleviated over time can be a critical source of diagnostic information. Look further into the symptoms and observe their variability before making a final diagnosis. Allow the patient time to process this information and for them to do some reading about these concepts. There are several good sources of information on PPD (see appendix) for patients to read that can help them understand the processes involved. When the provider and the patient work together over time, the diagnosis usually becomes apparent.

## Review Your Findings with the Patient

After completing the medical evaluation, whether or not the more detailed psychological interview is done, the clinician needs to inform the patient of the findings. The way this explanation is conducted can have a huge impact. Patients who understand and accept that they have a form of PPD are much more likely to have a better outcome. Clinicians who understand that psychophysiologic disorders are common can prepare their patients as part of their initial assessment with a statement such as this: "I have learned over the years that most symptoms can be caused by either medical disorders or stress, or some combination of the two. Therefore, I always investigate both of these possibilities to make sure that we understand what is causing the problems my patients have. That's critical in order to get the best treatment."

Demonstration of caring and empathy for the patient is key. Making empathic statements when hearing stories of stressful life events can help the patient see the magnitude of their own suffering and the link to psychophysiologic processes. "It must have been hard being put in between your parents like that. No wonder you had stomach aches then. I'm so sorry that happened to you." Or "It's common for sexually abused children to have physical symptoms like you did, especially when they are unable to tell anyone about it. It makes me sad for you. You deserved better." Encourage patients to feel empathy for themselves. Give them the opportunity to experience whatever feelings arise as they speak of earlier life experiences.

Even when clinicians understand that PPDs are common and not the fault of the patient, there is a tendency to stigmatize the patient with this diagnosis. Linking the onset of symptoms to the presence of significant stressful events is one way to help the clinician gain empathy for each patient. Once a structural process has been ruled out, it is essential to carefully explain the nature of a psychophysiologic disorder: doing this carefully will also build trust and communicate empathy. The next chapter reviews this in detail.

Many patients will have concerns about such a diagnosis, feeling that they are being told that their pain is not real, that it is "all in their head," that they are responsible for the pain, or that they are being blamed for it. Many patients hope to find they are suffering from a specific physical disorder that can be easily treated and cured—even though they probably have had several workups that have not done so. They are often disappointed to learn that they have "just" a psychophysiologic disorder, not a physical disease. But a diagnosis of PPD is good news—it's a real disorder that can be effectively treated without medications or surgery (Hsu, et. al., 2010; Abbass, et. al., 2005; Abbass, et. al., 2008; Abbass, et. al., 2009; Schechter and Smith, 2005; Burger, et. al., 2016; Lumley, et. al., 2017; Coughlin, 2006).

If you are comfortable in doing so, you might describe to your patients about times when you had pain caused by neural pathways. Or you might describe other patients you have seen who had good outcomes after getting this diagnosis.

## Table 2.3: Clues to the Diagnosis of PPD

- Occurrence of a significant number of PPDs in the past (Review of Symptoms lifetime checklist)
- History of adverse childhood events (ACE scale)
- Personality traits of self-criticism, self-sacrificing, perfectionism, need to please, and others (personality traits checklist)
- Onset of symptoms coincide with significant stressful life events (life trajectory interview)
- Symptoms are in a distribution pattern inconsistent with a structural disorder, such as symmetric or one whole side of the body, or the whole arm or leg
- Symptoms have persisted after normal healing would have occurred
- Symptoms shift from one location in the body to others
- Symptoms spread from one area to adjacent regions
- Symptoms are bilateral in distribution
- Symptoms occur due to social contagion
- Symptoms vary with time of day, place, or activity in discernible patterns
- Symptoms are absent with a certain activity or exercise, but then occur later in the day or the next day
- Symptoms often begin or occur in the middle of the night or upon awakening
- Symptoms are correlated with stressful situations or the anticipation of stressful situations, such as family visits or work stress
- Physical exam does not reveal clear objective signs of pathology; no evidence of injury and a normal neurological examination
- Light palpation elicits significant symptoms or results in unusual radiation of symptoms
- Lab studies and imaging reveal normal or "normative" findings, such as degenerative disc disease or bulging discs frequently found in patients without pain
- Symptoms are triggered in the office when discussing stressful events
- Symptoms are alleviated in the office when exposed to either cognitive-behavioral (see chapters 3 and 4) or emotion-focused sessions (chapters 5-8)

## CHAPTER 2 SUMMARY

- *Psychophysiologic disorders are very common in patients seeking medical care; have a high index of suspicion for them.*

- *PPDs typically occur in individuals with a history of adverse childhood events and certain personality traits and are usually triggered by stressful life events.*

- *PPDs are activated via learned neural pathways in the brain, in the absence of tissue damage.*

- *Establishing a culture in your patients of thinking about stress factors can make it easier to consider them in their visit.*

- *A trusting relationship and a thorough clinical evaluation are keys to a good PPD diagnosis.*

- *The diagnosis of a PPD can be made after a structural disorder is ruled out and a PPD is ruled in.*

CHAPTER 3

# Explaining Psychophysiologic Disorders

AFTER CONFIRMING that the patient suffers from PPD rather than a pathological process, the next step is to outline a treatment program, beginning with education. Many patients with PPDs have been incorrectly diagnosed with disorders that include significant tissue damage. Doctors have told others there is nothing wrong with them despite their significant, even overwhelming, symptoms. For years they have been in pain, and that pain has been aggravated by the fear of having a terrible disease or an unknown incurable condition. No wonder, then, that when they find out their condition is not dire, a significant number of patients see their symptoms quickly abate. Education and reassurance alone can improve or even reverse PPD symptoms, especially in patients on the left side of the PPD Causation Spectrum (see chapter 1), who have relatively more emotional resiliency and have experienced relatively less severe trauma in life. Once they know their condition is caused by learned neural pathways, is not debilitating, and is reversible, their fear, worry, and attention to their symptoms begin to subside. It is precisely the neural loop of fear-pain-fear that perpetuates PPD and education can start to alter these neural pathways.

You can tell your patient that if she understands her condition and believes it is PPD then it is likely that she will have the energy and confidence to take additional steps to resolve her symptoms. The more the patient understands and accepts the diagnosis, the more likely a rapid recovery, using the cognitive and behavioral interventions described in chapter 4, will be effective. Some have suggested that some of the approaches outlined in this book are merely a placebo effect. Placebo effects are often thought to be non-specific and able to help everyone to a small degree. However, when neural coding of expectations of chronic pain or other PPD symptoms is the underlying reason for the persistence of symptoms, changing that expectation (which is the definition of the placebo effect) can literally cure the disorder. The placebo effect has been shown to be very effective in certain conditions. In mild to moderate depression, placebo responses are equal to those of anti-depressants (Kirsch, 2010).

Another criticism of this approach is the emphasis on needing to believe that the diagnosis of PPD is correct, implying that this is akin to a religious conversion. However, in order to be successful in the treatment of PPD, a key component is the reduction of fear to decrease activation of the danger/alarm mechanism in the brain. It is difficult to reduce fear when the patient continues to hold the conviction that there is persistent, dangerous tissue damage in their body. Some cancer patients do not accept their diagnosis and may avoid potentially life-saving treatment. For patients with PPD, we believe it makes sense to accept that diagnosis in order to obtain the most effective treatment.

There are four major components of treatment for psychophysiologic disorders:

1) Education on the nature of the disorder
2) Reduction of the danger/alarm mechanisms of the brain
3) Making necessary changes in activities and life situations
4) Processing emotions that are linked to the symptoms

## Build the Therapeutic Relationship

Studies have shown that a trusting relationship between the clinician and patient accounts for much of the improvement seen in clinical settings (Safran, et. al., 2006). Take time to listen to your patients, affirm your understanding of their situations, and commit to helping them. These steps can create a strong bond, a therapeutic alliance. For most patients, no one has taken the time to listen and look at the symptoms carefully enough to really understand them—even though the impact of personal, family, and work stressors on patients' health has been emphasized in the training of health professionals for more than 100 years (Peabody, 1927; Stone, 1995).

Patient outcomes improve when the clinician and patient agree on the diagnosis and treatment (Starfield, 1981). This is particularly important with psychophysiologic disorders. Time spent helping patients understand the nature of PPD is an important positive step. We recognize that patients who present with multiple symptoms and who are on multiple medications can be challenging for health care providers on several levels. It is an act of great kindness and wisdom to take the time to look beneath the symptoms to the person under them who is suffering greatly and who, most likely, has suffered greatly in their life.

## Reviewing the Evidence

It is important to point out the specific evidence for the diagnosis of PPD. Patients with back or neck pain can be reassured that minor abnormalities seen on X-rays or MRIs are common and due to the normal process of aging; they do not represent pathologic processes. Show the patient data on the prevalence of degenerative discs, bulging discs, and herniated discs in asymptomatic people of varying ages (see table 2.2). Review instances where pain or other symptoms varied in severity or disappeared for some time to explain that they are due to neural pathways "turned on" and "turned off" by the brain. Explain the links between stressful life events that condition the brain and the body to be programmed for pain or other symptoms. Provide a list of this evidence for the patient to keep and review. It is often helpful to annotate this list with details that support this diagnosis, such as lists of symptoms, negative tests, and specific instances when symptoms were exacerbated.

I REVIEWED *this material with Elizabeth and answered her
questions. Elizabeth is relieved to know that there may be a
reason for her symptoms and asks what can be done about
it. It makes sense to her that the symptoms are not caused
by structural problems because they have shifted around so
much and her tests have been normal. She knows that she has
experienced a great deal of hurt and stress in her life and can
understand that this may have caused her brain to activate the
"danger" response that has produced her symptoms. She is
cautiously excited about a new treatment plan but still worried
that she won't get better.*

HERE IS THE EVIDENCE LIST FOR ELIZABETH:
- *Symptoms in many areas and in many organ systems*
- *No clear medical diagnosis despite physical
  examination and multiple workups*
- *Significant adverse childhood experiences*
- *Personality traits checklist consistent with those
  commonly held by PPD patients*
- *Onset and exacerbation of symptoms associated
  with significant stressful events*

### When There is Uncertainty

There often is some uncertainty in this diagnosis. It can
be difficult to prove with certainty that specific symptoms are
due to PPD. You can be quite certain the diagnosis is correct
if symptoms are entirely removed by cognitive-behavioral
exercises (see chapter 4) or by emotionally focused therapy
(chapters 5-8). But upon first hearing this diagnosis, many
patients are skeptical. Don't argue with them if they are not
ready to accept the diagnosis. Ask the patient to keep an open
mind while engaging in a treatment program or gathering more
evidence. At times, a patient may need more medical evaluations
to completely rule out other diagnoses. The diagnosis may
not be proven correct until the patient sees symptoms change
with different life events or disappear with psychotherapeutic
interventions.

In some patients, some of the symptoms are due to PPD and some are due to structural causes. In these situations, first treat symptoms that are more likely to be due to PPD and see how the patient responds. Later, you may be able to work on other symptoms as you learn more about them through more medical evaluations or by investigating their relationship to neural pathways (looking for relationships with stress or how symptoms vary over time).

PETER IS A BIT MORE SKEPTICAL. *He finds it hard to believe that his pain is caused by his brain when his other doctors and physical therapists have dignosed a structural problem. I review his MRI with him and the prevalence of MRI "abnormalities" in asymptomatic people of his age (see table 2.2). I also show him the MRI findings of patients who had PPD and recovered (with their permission). I point out that he has pain where his MRI is normal and that he had no pain while on the boat. I agree with him that it can be very difficult to believe that intense pain can be caused by the brain. I suggest that he keep an open mind as I continue to treat him. Since past treatments have not worked, he agrees to move forward with this approach.*

## Introduce Psychophysiologic Disorders as a Concept

Discuss the following with your patient. Symptoms are manifestations of an underlying process that must be investigated and explained. Whether the symptom is pain, anxiety, depression, fatigue, insomnia, diarrhea, urinary frequency, or anything else, it's either caused by tissue damage (a pathological process in the body), by neural pathways (a physiological process that can be reversed using psychological interventions), or a combination of the two. If all specific pathological processes that might be causative have been ruled out, the patient is suffering from a neural pathway problem. Symptoms due to neural pathways are real and can be at least as severe as symptoms caused by tissue damage. Tell patients that you understand their suffering and will work to the best of your ability to help them recover. As mentioned, listening carefully to the patient's story and taking their symptoms seriously is critical in treating patients with PPD.

## Explain Neural Pathways

The next step is to explain that neural pathways consist of thousands of brain cells that have formed connections, creating a network that activates specific thoughts, emotions, or actions. They are formed by a process of repetition and connection to specific outcomes or reinforcements (Kandel and Hawkins, 1992; Hawkins, et. al., 1983). Babies are born with innate pathways that govern suckling, turning towards sounds, being attracted to certain tastes, and many other actions. As they grow, the brains of children create thousands of neural pathways by learning cognitive skills such as speech, reading, and mathematics, as well as physical activities such as gestures, walking, riding a bicycle, and many more. Neural pathways mediate the majority of activities we engage in on a daily basis. These neural processes operate in the subconscious, which controls our bodily functions, such as breathing, heart rate, muscle tension, balance, and visual processing.

## Help Patients Understand the Role Of The Brain

Emotional reactions are also learned by life experiences and activated by our brains in response to new situations on an automatic basis (Feldman Barrett, 2017). Our brains also activate physical reactions in the body, such as pain or anxiety, in conjunction with strong emotions whether we are actually aware of the emotions or not. Patients with PPD can understand that the brain can activate these physical symptom pathways in response to either physical or emotional stimuli (Kross, et. al., 2011; Eisenberger, et. al., 2006). Most such stimuli occur on a subconscious level, and the patient becomes aware of the cause only when the reaction occurs in their body or their conscious mind (LeDoux, 1996; Damasio, 2000). With specific PPD symptoms, once the brain has established a neural pathway, they can be continuously or intermittently activated by ongoing subconscious psychological factors, by conditioned responses to certain stimuli, or simply by the neural expectation that they will continue to be activated. Over time, pain pathways can become more entrenched and activated regularly. However, these pathways can also be "turned off," and other non-painful neural pathways can be activated. This becomes obvious when pain and other symptoms occur one moment and disappear the next or when pain moves from one body area to another.

Help your patient understand the process by which pain pathways are formed in the brain. When an injury occurs to the body, nerve signals are transmitted to the interoceptive network of the brain that consists of many structures including the amygdala, anterior cingulate cortex, and other areas. Those structures then activate an alarm signal within milliseconds. This signal *causes* our sensation of physical pain and the simultaneous awareness of danger in the conscious brain. We must be able to feel pain to protect ourselves from further injury by, for instance, removing our hand from a hot stove and seeking appropriate treatment. People who have a complete lack of fear or the sense of danger can suffer significant injuries during the course of daily life.

However, pain does not occur with all physical injuries. Beecher interviewed soldiers who were injured in World War II, and the majority denied having pain (Beecher, 1951). A friend of mine told of seeing a man beaming with pride as he showed his wife a conch shell he'd found in the ocean, oblivious to many lacerations on his legs. Another friend of mine showed me a picture of his thumb after he had accidentally shot a nail into it. He had felt no pain and had driven himself to the hospital. Children who fall and skin their knee often cry, but many don't at all; and some only cry when they see a parent arrive with a worried expression on their face (which then activates the neural response of pain and tears).

When pain occurs, it causes muscle tension, changes in blood flow, and activation of catecholamines and the immune system. This process completes the construction of a new neural pathway, which will be stored like other learned behaviors or activities in the brain's memory. A doctor told me that as a young man he was injured in the Vietnam War in a firefight, sustaining shrapnel wounds to his left leg. He was airlifted to safety. After his return home and rehabilitation therapy, the pain in his leg went away. Twenty years later, he noticed the same type of pain in the same leg while walking outside and hearing the sound of a helicopter. The danger signal in his brain was triggered by the sound and activated the learned neural pathway and the leg pain.

Tell your patient that the danger signal can be activated by physical injury or also by emotional injury or threat. Studies have shown that emotional hurts trigger the same patterns as physical injuries. When volunteers were exposed to a mildly painful heat stimulus on their forearms, an fMRI showed activation of specific areas of the brain. When they were shown a picture of a romantic partner who had recently broken up with them, the fMRI scan showed that the same areas of the brain were activated (Kross, et. al., 2011). Doctors in Britain reported a case of a man who jumped off a scaffolding and felt severe pain when he saw his foot was impaled on a large nail. He was rushed to the hospital, sedated, and given intravenous pain medications. But when his shoe was removed, the nail was lodged between his toes, and there was no injury to his foot (Fisher, et. al., 1995). The brain can create severe pain when the danger signal is activated, even in the absence of tissue damage, but this pain is just as real.

The fact is that all pain is created by the brain. The same is true for anxiety, depression and other symptoms of PPD. The symptoms are a *message* that the brain is sending to us. When pain is caused by a physical injury, we are being "told" to attend to the injury. When the pain is caused by the brain in the absence of a physical injury, the meaning is vastly different, as would be the appropriate treatment.

When pain occurs, our conscious mind quickly attempts to figure out what is causing it and assesses the severity of the danger. Is it a matter of survival, a temporary nuisance, or something in between? The answer has a large effect on the pain. When pain is interpreted as being due to a serious physical injury or if it is overwhelming or leads to fear or helplessness (such as being unable to handle an important event or task), the pain tends to be exacerbated. People who respond to pain as if it's a catastrophe are more likely to develop chronic pain (Severeijns, 2001). A key in treating PPD is to accurately interpret the source of pain and control the conscious brain mechanisms that can turn off specific neural pain pathways. The more frequently a pain pathway is activated, the more it becomes a default mode. With treatment for PPD, patients learn to activate the "no pain" pathways to overcome this default mode. This is the neurological basis of recovery from PPD.

## Personalize the Information

It is helpful to explain to patients how these neurological processes developed in response to specific life events to create the particular PPD symptoms. Using the data obtained in the life trajectory interview (see appendix), the provider can link traumatic events to the onset and exacerbation of PPD symptoms. Explain that the brain activates an alarm signal to produce pain or fear in situations that are deemed to be unsafe. When we are exposed to stressful life events, our brains create pathways consisting of emotional memory. Neural pathways signifying danger that develop in childhood are particularly strong, including responses to events such as loss, abandonment, and physical, emotional, or sexual abuse. Many patients with PPD, however, have not experienced such obvious trauma but milder sorts of distress, as do most children to some degree. Children with a parent (or two) who are self-centered or who have a disabled or emotionally unstable sibling can fail to meet the needs of a sensitive child. This child often feels the need to be "perfect" to win praise or even have emotional needs recognized. Over time, such a child's brain learns to react to insults, injuries, and traumatic events with strong feelings and secondary physical anxiety.

This danger or anxiety signal can easily become activated by later stressful events, especially if they are emotionally similar. These "triggers" can activate old feelings, anxiety and fear pathways to create PPD symptoms. For example, a woman whose father frequently yelled at her developed headaches when a new boss began yelling at her in a similar fashion. The danger/ alarm mechanism was "primed" by her father and then later "triggered" by her boss. Another patient grew up in a family with an irresponsible younger sister, and the patient covered up for her to avoid her parents' anger. As an adult responsible for a large project on a tight deadline, she also covered up for an irresponsible colleague and subsequently developed widespread pain. In these situations, the pain is a message of danger being activated by the brain. Patients are often surprised by the revelation of such links.

Many events—including car accidents, surgery, or other traumas—can be triggers even if not emotionally similar to the priming events. A brain that has a sensitized danger signal can easily develop new symptom pathways with even relatively small insults, such as a minor car accident or a mild muscle sprain, especially if those injuries occur at the same time as other stressful life events. As mentioned, not all patients with PPD have had overtly abusive childhoods; everyone has the capacity to develop psychophysiologic disorders. Most people have had some sorts of psychophysiologic reactions in their lives. It is part of being human and how our brains and bodies are connected.

Through the joint discovery process you conduct, patients often develop a much deeper understanding of the relationship between the mind and the body and can begin to understand that their symptoms are caused by the brain's response to emotional trauma and threats: neural pathways rather than structural disorders (see table 3.1).

## Results of Patient Education

By taking the time to listen to the patient's life story, the clinician can learn about the basis for their PPD symptoms. By carefully explaining the neurophysiological basis of PPD, the clinician will also help the patient understand that PPD is real and can be reversed. Patients will feel respected, and their symptoms will be validated. That understanding can decrease fear and worry and the pain that accompanies those emotions and increase their ability to heal by strengthening them to face emotional challenges. Several patients have told me: "I'm so glad that the pain is not in my head, but that it's in my brain."

A woman with chronic back pain said this after education about psychophysiologic illness:

> "I HAVE HAD *chronic back pain for over 20 years. It has caused significant limitations in every aspect of my life. I have had three back surgeries to try to reverse it, but despite claims of technical successes, the pain has continued. My third surgery, a three-level fusion, was 21 months ago. I have spent this time trying every therapy in the book, anything and everything to get out of enormous and unrelenting back pain. With no success....*"

> "*My doctor sent me the link to your website 6 days ago. I went to it the next day and considered the possibility that yes, maybe this could apply to me. I came back a day later to read all the material more seriously and realized: absolutely, this describes me to a "T." With that shift in belief, the back pain subsided—almost like "poof!" It went from a seven to a one on the pain scale, to off the pain scale onto a "discomfort" scale. I believe this was totally due to the complete shift in my belief system—no halfway for me. It came from a total realization: this is me. Then, another big change occurred. Once I really "got it" that there is nothing structurally wrong with my back, on the fourth day, I started walking. I could barely walk around the building at first, but I kept up a steady mantra of "I can walk; I am OK." And there I was taking a pleasant walk.*"

> "*...what a day-and-night difference—from crippled, fearful, bewildered, discouraged, bordering on despair —to on my way to regaining my life.*"

It should be noted that a relatively small proportion of patients have this kind of response to education. For most patients, understanding that they have a PPD is necessary, but not sufficient to eliminate the symptoms.

## Managing Mixed PPD/Pathological Conditions

Many patients have elements of a PPD and a structural disorder. These individuals can be treated with a combination of medical and psychophysiologic treatments. Those with pure PPD can be treated with the treatment described in the next chapters.

Some people with mixed presentations will resist the suggestion that some of their symptoms are due to psychologically based brain processes. Be patient. Over time the true nature of the disorders will become evident. If the symptoms change in ways that do not conform to pathologic disorders, if symptoms improve or worsen in relation to psychological or social stimuli, if further medical evaluations do not identify a structural etiology, and if medical treatments are ineffective or worsen the symptoms, the diagnosis of PPD becomes clearer.

I recently saw a patient who had paresthesias and muscle twitching in several different areas of his body. He had an extensive medical workup which was normal, which made it clear that these symptoms were due to PPD. However, he also had a nerve-like pain radiating down one arm and had a bulging disc between the corresponding cervical vertebrae. After careful history and physical examination, as described in chapter 2, it was still somewhat difficult to be certain if the arm pain was due to PPD or not. After much consideration, he had surgery to remove the offending disc. Following the surgery, the arm pain and the other symptoms were markedly improved. But two weeks later, all of the symptoms returned. Thus, it became obvious that his symptoms, including the arm pain, were due to PPD. This realization led this patient to be certain of his diagnosis and using the techniques described in the next chapter, he was able to dramatically reduce his symptoms.

The prevalent paradigm in medicine gives little credence to the power of the mind-body connection. It is our hope that advances in neurology, psychology, and medicine begin to become more widely known and more patients will accept the concept of psychophysiologic contributions to symptoms.

## Table 3.1: **Key Points in Explaining PPD to Patients**

1. **Empathize:** "That sounds horrible. I can't imagine how awful this has been."

2. **Ally:** "I want to help. We need to work together to find answers. What has been tried is clearly not working."

3. **Explain pain:** "Let me tell you about the latest scientific facts about pain (or other symptoms) that most people and many doctors aren't aware of yet."

4. **Personalize:** "Here's how these ideas may apply to your situation."

5. **Offer hope:** "Given all of this information, I believe there is hope for you to get better, rather than simply cope with your symptoms."

## Sample Script for Brief Education on Pain Caused by PPD

(Alter the message accordingly for other symptoms of PPD.)

The pain of neural pathway disorders is very real and can be quite severe. All pain occurs in the brain, whether it is due to a structural disorder or not. Pain occurs when our brain activates an alarm or danger signal. Both physical injuries and emotional injuries activate the same danger signal, which triggers pain. People with pain do not always have physical injuries (and people with injuries do not always have pain). When pain occurs (whether due to an injury or a neural pathway process), the brain learns the neural pathways associated with that pain. These neural pathways can become persistent, can be turned off, or can come and go depending on whether the danger signal in the brain is activated. People exposed to stressful life events are more likely to have a danger/alarm mechanism that is sensitive and activates pain and other symptoms. Pain frequently occurs due to neural pathways (PPD). It's part of how our brains and bodies work.

## CHAPTER 3 SUMMARY

- *Education about PPD can allay fears and lead to improvements or resolution of symptoms in some patients.*

- *PPDs are common, and most people have them at some time.*

- *PPDs are caused by learned neural pathways and are not associated with tissue damage.*

- *The symptoms of PPD are real, not imagined, and are due to physiological activation of the alarm mechanism in the brain.*

- *PPD is reversible with treatment.*

CHAPTER 4

# Cognitive and Behavioral Interventions

MANAGING PPD BEGINS WITH EXPLAINING the diagnosis (see chapter 3). If there is resistance to the diagnosis, spend more time in discussion and investigation. Observe closely what brings on and relieves symptoms and the timing of these events. By learning what emotions or circumstances trigger symptoms in each patient, you can gain more insight into how the brain turns symptoms on and off. An upper back massage may trigger pain in the lower back or pelvis, a phone call from a relative may cause a stomach ache, or thinking about the absence of pain can lead to its appearance. Pain may disappear when complete attention to an important task is required or when relaxing. The more the patient understands and accepts the diagnosis, the more likely they will respond to cognitive and behavioral interventions. If a patient is ambivalent about the diagnosis, you can initiate treatment and the patient will often become more convinced as they see these connections and as symptoms abate. But do not proceed with the following interventions if there is strong resistance to the diagnosis. Instead, spend more time on investigating the mind-body connections with the patient, or consider proceeding to the emotion-focused therapeutic approach outlined in chapters 5-8.

## Basis for Use of Cognitive Behavioral Interventions

Treatment of PPD includes cognitive and behavioral interventions. If patients accept the diagnosis that there is nothing physically wrong, their pain and the accompanying tension, fear, withdrawal, and helplessness can be reduced. Then they can work on reducing the automatic, natural, fearful reactions to pain and other PPD symptoms that are reinforcing the neural pathways that are the current cause of the symptoms (Gracely and Schweinhardt, 2015). This requires your patients to alter how they view the symptoms and how they respond to them.

Even though many of the cognitive and behavioral interventions described below are similar to standard cognitive-behavioral therapy (CBT) for pain, there are some important distinctions. Most patients receiving CBT for pain do not have a careful evaluation to search for PPD and therefore all pain is treated as being due to structural disorders. Because of this, the primary goal of standard CBT for chronic pain is to cope with the pain in order to manage it better. Finally, CBT treatments typically do not address underlying emotional conditions. Indeed, meta-analyses (van Dessel, et. al., 2014) point to only small effects from standard CBT in somatoform disorders. The goal of the following interventions for patients with PPD is to eliminate, rather than cope with, the pain and other PPD symptoms. This distinction is critical to the success of this approach.

## Symptom Tracking: Noticing Antecedents

Pain and other psychophysiologic symptoms are fueled by a fear of being damaged or hurt. Many healthcare providers have told PPD patients that there is something wrong with their bodies, that they will have pain and other symptoms for the rest of their lives. They are often told to avoid physical activity. It may take several sessions for patients to fully accept the diagnosis of PPD and let go of the idea that their symptoms are due to a degenerated or bulging disc or a damaged nerve. Encourage them to notice when they are better or worse, particularly in relation to stressful or emotional events. Look for instances when pain or other symptoms shift, move, or vary in specific movements or situations. Identify when pain or other symptoms are absent to help show that the symptoms *can* go away. Even though you have diagnosed them with PPD, many need repeated reassurance and as much evidence as possible to fully convince themselves that they do, in fact, have PPD.

AFTER THE FIRST VISIT, *I ask Elizabeth to pay attention to times when her symptoms are better or worse. That week, she noticed that when her co-workers were critical of her, she got a headache. On one occasion when her boyfriend called, her arms and hands had burning pain for several minutes. I congratulate her on recognizing these connections. This is a significant step in her recovery. In addition, I remind her that when she told me about the prior sexual abuse, she had tension in her jaw and neck. After this review, Elizabeth is more convinced that emotional factors are central to her difficulties. She feels some relief but sighs as she leaves the office, though she still feels overwhelmed.*

PETER HAS NOTED THAT *his back pain gets better and worse at times. He has little back pain when he is sitting at home or in the car, but has significant pain when sitting at work. I point out that pain due to structural causes is unlikely to have this kind of variation. He thought that this was due to the difference in chairs. However, changing his work chair has not made a difference. This realization helps Peter to understand this much better. He smiles when I tell him that he is going to get better.*

## Reappraisal of PPD Symptoms and Reduction of Fear

When pain or other symptoms occur, the patient can begin to retrain their reactions. A first step is to reappraise the symptoms as being due to a psychophysiologic process that will resolve over time, not due to something seriously wrong in the body. Conscious affirmation of this fact helps to allay the fear response.

Emphasize to the patient that fear is the driving force behind PPD. The brain is trying to alert the patient to danger. If we touch a hot stove, the pain teaches us not to do so again. If we break a leg, the pain tells us to avoid walking on that leg and to seek treatment. In psychophysiologic disorders, the pain and other symptoms alert us to emotional dangers in our lives— and these can be a combination of prior traumatic events, current stressful situations, and the stress produced by the symptoms themselves. It takes courage to face fears and move ahead despite them. Reassure, encourage, and congratulate your patient for her efforts. This work can be very difficult and require great perseverance. If patients begin to worry whether they will ever recover, this worry itself can increase the danger signal and delay recovery. If patients become impatient that they are not getting better as quickly as they would like, this impatience also becomes an impediment to recovery. Encourage them to relax in the knowledge that they are not damaged and are going to get better, although you cannot give them a time frame for their recovery.

Over time, patients can begin to view their PPD symptoms as ways that their brain is trying to protect them—and eventually realize that they don't actually need this protection and decline the brain's warning signal. For example, their brain interprets certain places, situations, movements, or positions as dangerous, thus creating pain or other symptoms at those times. The brain is interpreting normal sensations that it receives from that painful body part as if it were an injury, thus producing pain. Our job is to work with patients to reassure them and teach them methods of reversing these learned neural pathways.

## Conceiving of PPD as a Bully

I frequently use this analogy to help patients in their recovery. Psychophysiologic symptoms are like bullies that use fear as a means of control. Children who are bullied constantly fear being trapped by their tormentor. Pain, anxiety, depression, or fatigue due to PPD operates similarly: those who suffer from this syndrome worry about their symptoms; doubt they will ever get better; feel helpless and victimized; and live with guilt, shame, and self-pity. PPD symptoms are reinforced by the constant worry and fear they create. Patients with chronic pain and other conditions are often told to keep a diary of how often the symptoms occur and how severe they are, but such diaries have been shown to be counterproductive because the increased focus on painful symptoms can cause them to worsen (Ferrari and Russell, 2010; Ferrari, 2015; Ferrari and Louw, 2013).

To stop bullying, the victim can fight back. Encourage your patients to stop allowing pain or other symptoms to rule them, to instead take control and realize they can overcome the symptoms. They can also just stop paying so much attention to the bully, to stop being afraid of the symptoms. If the bully calls you a name, your response can be, "That's a good one. Got any other names to call me?" It is often very hard to completely ignore or "not care" about pain and other symptoms, but as patients learn to separate from the symptoms, worry less about them, and ignore them without fear, they are training their brain to eliminate the neural pathways of pain. They can practice smiling or even laughing at the symptoms as they understand them and gain freedom from fear, which helps resolve PPD symptoms. Such work fosters assertiveness, which is often missing in patients with PPD due to factors such as early life adversity and certain personality traits as discussed above.

## Use Top-Down Cognitive Interventions

At times, patients with chronic PPD symptoms experience themselves as helpless victims. The symptoms can function as a repetition of abuse by a powerful controlling person in their past. This re-experiencing of trauma activates brain alarm systems that lead to the perpetuation of symptoms. As the patient learns to retrain their cognitive reactions to pain and other PPD symptoms, they can begin to move forward with confidence. Urge them to replace helpless and fearful thoughts with messages such as "I am healthy and strong" and "There is nothing wrong with me." Encourage patients to speak directly to their symptoms, often aloud, with phrases like "Pain—you're nothing," "You can't hurt me anymore," "I am not stopping my activities or giving in to you anymore," "I am powerful and am removing your control over me," and "I am not afraid of you."

These affirmations are akin to the "fighting back" approach to a bully. We all know that we can use our brain to control our body functions, such as when we need to delay urination or slow our breathing. When patients fully understand PPD and begin to believe that they can get better, they can begin to feel more powerful and in control. Changing the internal dialogue can override the damaging effects of helplessness and victimization. A recent study found that affirmations activate the ventromedial prefrontal cortex, a part of the brain that can attenuate the danger responses of the amygdala and other limbic structures (Falk, et. al., 2015).

## Behavioral Interventions

Pain and other symptoms can be conditioned responses to stimuli such as changes in the weather, foods, light, sounds, and many other things. Some researchers now recommend learning to defuse triggers to migraine headaches rather than avoiding them (Martin, 2010). Recent studies have shown that the effects of weather on back and joint pain are not demonstrable (Steffens, et. al., 2014; Ferreira, et. al., 2016). Avoiding triggers can lead to increased fear and helplessness. Exposure to triggers with the knowledge that they are activating the brain to create symptoms rather than causing symptoms due to tissue damage can lead to abatement of PPD symptoms. For example, patients can begin to eat certain foods that have triggered their symptoms in the past as they tell their brain the food is safe and won't bother them. The same is true with sitting, standing, walking, bending, or other physical activities previously avoided. When these triggers are challenged with confidence, the symptoms will wane over time and patients can develop the healing states of equanimity and optimism as they gradually move towards recovery.

AT PETER'S NEXT VISIT, *he tells me that he is more active although he is still having significant pain. He notes that he always gets pain when he bends over toward his right side. This makes him doubt the diagnosis of a PPD. I congratulate him on his progress. Being more active despite pain is an important step in his recovery process.*

*I then ask if he is willing to investigate this in the office. I explain that this pain is a learned response; that bending to the right causes pain because it activates his brain to create pain, not because his body is damaged. I explain that he can "unlearn" that response.*

*I ask him to stand up and assume a powerful posture (feet spread apart, chest and head up, arms up and hands clenched), repeat a set of positive affirmations, and then bend to the right to see if he can alter this response. I coach him to say: "I am strong and healthy. There is nothing wrong with my back. Pain, I'm not afraid of you. Brain, relax. I'm fine, and I'm going to bend my back, and it will be fine." He then bends to that side. The pain is there, but slightly less than before. I ask him to repeat this process several times. Each time, the pain becomes a bit less. This process will eventually alter the pathways, and his pain will be decreased or eliminated* (see table 4.1).

"Powerful" postures have been shown to increase testosterone, reduce cortisol, and increase the pain threshold (Bohns and Wiltermuth, 2012; Carney, et. al., 2010).

## Table 4.1: Empowerment Exercise: Affirmations

### Educational: Understand

I'm healthy; I'm strong; there is nothing wrong with me.
I'm in charge; I can do what I want.

### Behavioral: Activate

Pain, symptoms, fearful thoughts: You're nothing.
I'm not afraid of you.
I don't need you; you can't hurt me anymore.

### Moving on: Calm

I'm going to ignore you and focus on what I want and need to do.
I am fine; I'm OK; I'll be fine.
I am safe and not in danger.
I'm retraining my brain every day.
I'm committed to my recovery.
I will find time for myself to enjoy life and move forward.

## Sample Script for Reducing PPD Symptoms

When pain or other symptoms occur, take a deep breath and remind yourself that there is nothing seriously wrong with your body. You are healthy, and the symptoms will subside soon. Tell your subconscious mind that it can now stop producing the symptoms. Do this with conviction, out loud or silently. Reframe the pain or other neural pathway symptoms as sensations that are not harming you. Take a deep breath and calm yourself. Remind yourself that you are safe and not in danger. Focus on things that you need to do in your life right now. Congratulate yourself on the steps you are taking to bring about recovery, even if symptoms persist for the time being.

## Sample Script For Reducing PPD Triggers

When you encounter any triggers to the symptoms (such as positions, places, movements, foods, weather changes, etc.) or any stressful situations, stop and take a deep breath. Remind your mind that this activity or situation will gradually cease to cause any symptoms or problems. For example, if you are bending over, remind yourself, "This will not cause any back problems. My back is healthy and strong, and I can do this without worrying about hurting myself." Understand that your body is healthy and that you can get better by not allowing your mind to produce symptoms. Relax and breathe in order to decrease fear. Repeat positive phrases about yourself, your body, and your recovery when you encounter any of your triggers until your brain stops activating PPD symptoms. The goal of this process is to reduce fear while doing the triggering activities, whether the symptoms occur or not. By reducing fear and continuing to challenge the triggers the neural pathways will be altered.

## Meditation and Mindfulness Practice

Meditation techniques are often effective in reducing fear. Patients can direct their attention to their breathing to practice calming the danger centers of the brain. As they practice this, patients can learn there is no immediate danger and they are safe. Mindfulness meditation is a method of altering brain responses to inputs from internal and external sources. These techniques have been refined during more than 2,500 years of practice and teaching (Kabat-Zinn, 1990; Goldstein, 2013). Mindfulness practice does not intend to distract the practitioner from brain inputs—including pain, thoughts, and emotions—but seeks to attend to these inputs with acceptance and less reactivity. This practice can be extremely valuable as a way of noticing internal states and separating from them. When PPD symptoms occur, one can begin to notice these sensations as "just sensations" in the body or as "peculiar sensations" that are not harmful. One can practice observing the sensation with curiosity, rather than reacting with fear, and recognizing the sensation as being produced by the brain. Mindfulness does not proscribe trying to make the pain go away, but facing the symptoms and feeling them without reacting. This directly and powerfully reduces fear and takes the fuel away from PPD symptoms.

Mindfulness practice is a potent way to deal with thoughts that undermine recovery. As with physical sensations, the process of mindful awareness is to notice thoughts with interest and without fear. Most PPD patients have a variety of fearful, intrusive, and repetitive thoughts. Examples include, "I'll never get better," "I must not be doing this correctly," "I'm too damaged already," and "I'm not good enough" (or smart enough, strong enough or persistent enough). Patients can train themselves to observe their thoughts, accept them as "just thoughts," and watch them pass. It is useful to explain to patients that such thoughts are common in most people and seen in almost all people with PPD.

Ask patients to practice noticing their physical sensations and thoughts in a mindful way by using the steps outlined below.

1. I'm noticing this physical sensation or this thought. That's interesting.
2. This sensation or thought is caused by my brain.
3. I can observe this sensation or thought without worry. It is just a peculiar sensation or just a thought.
4. It will pass or shift.
5. I am OK.
6. I will take a breath and watch for what arises next.

*Mindfulness*

This process is repeated throughout the day as patients learn that they can tolerate their thoughts and sensations, accept that they arise, and focus on observing with less reactivity. As patients practice recognizing these thoughts and feelings and continually react to them with dispassionate interest and calmness, they are training their brain away from the fear feedback loop. I urge them to do this many times per day, using shortcut phrases, like "Oh, that's my brain; I'm OK" or "This is just a thought, it will pass."

AT A FOLLOW-UP VISIT, *Elizabeth noted that some of her symptoms were constant but others came and went. She worried that some structural disorder was causing the constant pains in her head and neck. Since one doctor had told her that she had degenerative discs in her neck, she found it hard to believe that all her symptoms were caused by PPD.*

*I asked her to sit upright, close her eyes, and open her mind to a new way of looking at her symptoms. We started with mindful awareness of the breath, simply following the breath without trying to change it, observing it, and letting each breath go to focus on the next. Then I asked her to turn her attention to her head and follow the sensations there in the same way— observing them as if watching clouds in the sky, noticing them with less fear and less worry about the cause. I suggested that she notice any subtle changes in the sensations in her head for several minutes, i.e., noticing the sensations without trying to make them change, just attending to them in a kind way, not caring if the pain increases or decreases or stays the same, just watching to see if they change in any way, but not fearing them, and knowing that there is nothing wrong with her body, that the sensations are being caused by her brain. Then I asked her to focus again on her breath. Following that, I suggested that she use the same methods of mindful awareness on sensations in her hands; feeling these sensations and recognizing that these sensations are being interpreted by her brain as not unpleasant as she does not have pain there; as it's up to the brain how any sensations are being interpreted. Then I asked her to return to noticing sensations in her head once again. Again taking a few minutes to notice any sensations, knowing there is nothing wrong, but not caring at all right now if the sensations become more pleasant or more unpleasant as it doesn't matter, as she doesn't try to make the sensations go away, but she just attends to them with kindness towards herself. Towards the end of the exercise, I asked her to notice any bodily sensations in her neck in the same fashion as described above, observing without fear or worry, just noticing any sensations with interest and with less reactivity. We ended by returning her attention to the breath and inviting her to offer herself kindness.*

*Elizabeth reported that at first the head and neck pain was constant and got worse for a minute or so. But then, as she let go of some of her worries about the pain, it began to shift. When she was paying attention to the breath or the neck, the head pain vanished. A few minutes later, the neck pain also went away. Towards the end of the exercise, she noted pain in her lower back, but that quickly went away when she paid attention to it without fear. Then she suddenly said, "Now I just got a pain in my chest." I replied that this is typical of PPD that sensations shift from one spot to another, but that they will eventually go away. I suggested that she use her new ability to notice the chest pain without fear. After a while, that sensation went away as well.*

Teaching mindfulness to patients with PPD is both a diagnostic and therapeutic tool. It allows the provider and the patient to see that the symptoms are transient, not due to structural causes, gives the patient a clear demonstration of the true nature of the symptoms and provides a powerful tool for recovery. As Elizabeth learned to apply mindful awareness to her symptoms, she began to train her brain in the process of unlearning her pain.

Students of mindfulness will recognize this exercise as a variant of the "body scan." You can use this approach to examine and release tension or anxiety anywhere in the body. Mindfulness practice has been shown to reduce pain and for most people with PPD is a critical component of a treatment program (Grossman, et. al., 2007). However, I would emphasize that these techniques can have dramatic effects when applied to a patient who has the understanding and conviction that their symptoms are caused by PPD. When applied to people who believe they have a structural disorder causing their pain, those beliefs tend to undermine the ability to truly disregard the physical sensations and keep the patient in a state of fear that allows persistence of pain. A recent study comparing mindfulness to cognitive-behavioral therapy for low back pain showed that these two interventions were equivalent, and that the effects waned after one year (Cherkin, et. al., 2016). However, those patients were not assessed for, nor informed, about PPD.

## Compassion for Self

In addition to present moment awareness, mindfulness practice encourages participants to be kind and loving towards themselves and others in their lives. Practicing kindness to oneself is a critical component of healing in PPD. Due to trauma and neglect in childhood, PPD sufferers are likely to engage in excessive hyper-vigilance, people-pleasing behaviors, and self-criticism. They may have a great deal of buried, guilt-laden anger or even rage toward primary care providers, siblings or abusers. These processes typically occur in those who were subjected as children to excessive criticism, conditional acceptance, and more severe forms of abuse from first degree relatives. They cause one to react with strong feelings, anxiety and fear to stressful life events, whether due to emotional threats or to physical threats due to pain. When they react to current stressful situations, they are also reacting to earlier life stresses with reactivation of the same intense feelings. Because of this guilt and chronic childhood neglect, such individuals often have difficulty in being sympathetic to themselves. They may feel that they don't deserve to be cared for and loved. They often have little sympathy or have shut off feelings towards the child that grew up in their shoes (i.e., their own self).

Common internal processes that activate and perpetuate PPD include self-critical messages. Individuals who were criticized, bullied, or abused have often internalized those negative messages due to guilt about the anger toward the perpetrator. During times of adversity, such as when pain or other symptoms of PPD (including anxiety or depression) occur, patients often "hear" critical messages, such as "You are a loser," "This is all your fault," "You'll never get better," "You are not worth it," and other similar thoughts. We encourage our patients to consider these messages as coming from an internal bully and use the mindfulness techniques as described above. Once they realize that these thoughts are caused by a learned sense of self as inadequate due to prior negative experiences, they can begin to see that they don't need to be believed.

Another approach to PPD symptoms arises from the understanding that part of the reason for the symptoms is a lack of compassion towards oneself. Therefore, when pain or other PPD symptoms occur, the patient can take a moment to direct compassion and kindness to the symptom. This offers a softening of resistance that allows the neural pathways of pain to release.

For a significant number of people, providing education and teaching these cognitive and behavioral skills will create improvements or even resolution of PPD symptoms. However, these interventions do not necessarily address the core issues that have created the symptoms, the intense conflicted emotions that have typically not been identified, experienced, or processed (see chapters 5-8 for a detailed examination of these processes).

If a patient can visualize herself as a child who is in danger and afraid or hurt, she can often access feelings of sadness and loss. Ask the patient to give that child soothing messages out loud (such as "You didn't deserve to be treated this way," "You are now safe," and "I will protect you and love you,") and imagine holding and hugging that child. Then the patient can image soothing her current self. It may be helpful to have another person offer these loving and protective messages to the patient, or have the patient imagine getting these messages from a kind relative or friend or even from her own self as a child.

Some people who have difficulty generating compassion for themselves can imagine a child they care about—perhaps a child of their own—being in their past fearful situation they experienced as a child. Most patients with PPD will recoil at having their own children experience their own childhood. Chris Germer (2009) and Kristen Neff (2011) have written self-help guides to increasing self-compassion that are good resources for patients on this topic.

Another component of healing is forgiveness. Forgiveness does not imply forgetting what happened. It simply asserts that the issue will not continue to dominate one's life and one's mind, preventing one from being emotionally "hijacked" by past events. It has often been said that maintaining a grudge is like "swallowing poison and expecting the other person to die." It is a letting go of anger and hurt. Many patients have found that when they were able to forgive themselves for things they regretted, they were able to recover. It is important to address these issues in most PPD patients. Many patients have guilt about things that were outside of their control and can be counseled to realize that they actually did nothing wrong. In other situations, patients made mistakes and you can work with them to realize that they did the best they could at the time and work towards self-forgiveness. See *Forgive for Good* (Luskin, 2002) for more details.

Those who have been in pain a long time or who have experienced traumatic events tend to feel unsafe all the time. Ask your patients to take time each day to remind themselves that they are not in danger, take a deep breath, and move ahead. A patient of mine found that this simple practice of frequent reminders to himself that he was safe and not in danger was the most powerful component of his recovery from chronic pain.

I ASKED ELIZABETH TO *"go back"* to a moment in time *when she was hurt or in danger and see if she could feel compassion for the little girl or younger woman that was her. She immediately returned to a time in her life when she had been sexually abused and began to cry. After a couple of minutes, I asked her to imagine her grown self "going" (across time and space) to the younger Elizabeth to comfort her, hold her, and speak to her. She voiced (out loud) caring messages to the girl saying, "This is not your fault. You have done nothing wrong. You will get through this, and you're going to be OK. I will love you and protect you. You are a good person, and you are loved." This process allowed her to express sadness and grief, reduce guilt, and access compassion. Elizabeth noted that her neck muscles were more relaxed and that she felt "lighter."*

## Expressive Writing

There are some relatively simple interventions that medical and mental health providers can use to help patients begin to recognize and address emotional issues. A number of expressive writing exercises can be quite helpful. James Pennebaker has published several studies showing the power of writing in an unstructured way about significant emotional issues (Pennebaker, 1990; Pennebaker, 2004). With regard to physical symptoms, Lumley and colleagues have conducted studies demonstrating that expressive writing can be effective in asthma, fibromyalgia, and rheumatoid arthritis (Gillis, et. al., 2006; Norman, et. al., 2004; Smyth, et. al., 1999). Pennebaker asked individuals to take 15-20 minutes each day for several days and write extemporaneously about issues that were troubling to them. *Unlearn Your Pain* has a series of specific writing exercises designed to address emotional issues in people with PPD (Schubiner and Betzold, 2016). For example, patients can be encouraged to write an unsent letter to people who have been in their life (whether or not that person is still alive or part of their life) as a way of expressing thoughts and feelings that they have not been able to state directly. This technique allows one to express powerful feelings without regard to any consequences. The letter is not sent and may be destroyed as a symbolic way of letting the feelings go. Another technique is to create dialogues or conversations between the patient and another person or entity. These allow one to explore important issues by both "speaking" the truth and "hearing back" from another. Many of my patients have created dialogues between themselves and their pain (or other PPD symptoms). If a patient allows himself to explore the issue, he often discovers important lessons about why the symptoms are there and what they need to do to let them go (Schubiner and Betzold, 2016). After each of these writing exercises, we suggest the patient write a letter to himself to reflect on the issues that arose.

PETER WROTE A SERIES *of unsent letters, including ones to his father, his mother, his boss, and his son. As he did this, he saw how much anger he had towards all these people and felt lighter after expressing this anger. In addition, he realized how much he blamed himself for many things that had happened in his life. He felt particularly guilty for the problems his son had encountered, and he felt that if he were a better father, his son wouldn't have the problems he was now facing.*

*At his next visit, I was able to explain to him that his anger was justified and that expressing it in writing was healthy. I mention that he might also want to focus on forgiveness in future unsent letters as a way of letting go of the anger. I was also able to help him see that his guilt was not fully warranted, that he was the best father to his son that he could be, and that self-blame can be a significant contributor to his back pain. I asked him to consider having a talk with his son about these issues. He was making a great deal of progress in being more active. He had started biking and even began jogging again. He noted that his pain was much better. He felt that he was on the right path and was going to make a full recovery.*

### Emotional Awareness

Another intervention is to ask patients to begin to notice emotions as they occur. Emotions including anger that are suppressed or not recognized serve to activate the danger signal that triggers PPD symptoms. People with PPD tend to suppress and avoid emotions. It is very common for symptoms of pain or anxiety to develop when life events trigger emotions such as fear, anger, guilt, and grief. At these times, if patients can stop and look for underlying emotions as triggers for symptoms, they are often able to identify them, then allow the emotion to be felt and experienced, rather than blocking it or avoiding it. Often this provides patients with insight and understanding about the significant emotions underlying physical or psychological symptoms. In addition, experiencing and expressing emotions may attenuate or relieve current PPD symptoms. As will be described in subsequent chapters, emotional therapeutic processes are effective in addressing issues that caused PPD. When clinicians help patients identify and normalize their emotional reactions and create a safe environment for them, patients typically gain significant relief from PPD symptoms. It is important to explain to patients that they often may not recognize any particular thoughts or emotions when PPD symptoms occur. This is because those symptoms are often due to the learned patterns of neural pathways that have become engrained in the brain.

ELIZABETH WAS ASKED TO *pay attention to times when she notices any of her symptoms and see if she can recognize any feelings that underlie the symptoms. At her next visit, she stated that when her boyfriend texted her to tell her that he would not have dinner with her because he was going out with his friends, she began to have abdominal pain and a burning sensation in her hands. As she reflected on this, she realized that she felt hurt and abandoned as well as angry. She chose to soothe her hurt feelings, as she had learned to do in the exercise where she soothed herself as a child. And she allowed herself to feel the anger towards her boyfriend. As the anger rose, she noted that the stomach pain went away, yet the burning in her hands continued. She suddenly felt the urge to hit her boyfriend, and she blurted out: "Just go to hell." At that moment, the burning in her hands began to lessen. She immediately wrote several pages of her thoughts and feelings about the situation. When she was done, the burning in her hands was gone. She agreed to see a counselor who specializes in helping people deal with deeply held emotions, as she began to understand that accessing these feelings would be an important part of her recovery.*

### Examining Life Situations

Individuals with PPD are often in life situations that perpetuate distress and negative emotions. In addition, those with PPD are often non-assertive and self-devaluing and land in situations that create similar emotional reactions to those of the past. As part of their recovery, many will find it necessary to make changes in some of their relationships or life situations. Many people with PPD feel victimized and helpless. You may be able to help them stand up for themselves and feel more powerful, in control of their lives, confident, and feel better about themselves. If they are in a relationship that is abusive or dangerous, they may need to seek safety, rather than challenging their abuser. However, in certain situations, the ability to speak up or take action to make changes can be a critical component of recovery from psychophysiologic disorders.

ELIZABETH HAS SOME IMPORTANT *decisions to make with regard to her current boyfriend. Peter may be able to talk to his son about their relationship and work towards understanding and connection.*

### Resume Life

Patients who have the courage to live their lives as fully as possible, gradually increasing their activity and not allowing the symptoms to stop them from getting out of bed or going to work or school are taking powerful steps to reverse PPD. This is known as "outcome independence"—defining success as separate from having more or less symptoms. They can begin to live each day without fear of pain or other PPD symptoms. By engaging in more activities even if pain or other symptoms are present, they are altering their neural pathways. Part of recovery includes an increased focus on living rather than on the illness. The neural networks activated by exercise, connection to others, spirituality, engaging in work or hobbies, and creating awe-inspiring experiences (such as may occur in nature, prayer, meditation) directly activate brain regions that counteract those connected to fear and pain. Play and laughter are potent antidotes to psychophysiologic disorders and should be encouraged. They can be integral components of healing (Brown and Vaughan, 2009).

There is no set time frame for recovery from PPD. Liberated by the sudden realization that there is nothing physically wrong with them, some patients get better quickly. Others recover over several months as they incorporate the cognitive and behavioral components of treatment. Some have periods of few or no symptoms alternating with significant or severe symptoms. For some, the path to recovery is longer. It is critical for the health care provider to remain positive, reassuring, and encouraging throughout the process of recovery. While some patients find success with diagnosis, education, and affirmations, mindfulness is more effective for others, and some require emotion-focused techniques.

For those patients in whom the symptoms persist, some of the above techniques can actually become counterproductive if the patient is putting pressure on themselves to get better and focusing too much on the symptoms. In these cases, it is often necessary to focus less on their recovery and more on resuming their life, despite the persistence of symptoms. Many studies have shown that the keys to health include positive social connections and meaning and purpose in life. Therefore, it is often more important to focus on those issues, rather than the symptoms or their recovery efforts.

## Structuring Office Visits

How can medical or mental health clinicians accomplish some of these interventions? Many practitioners have little time to work with patients with PPD. However, it does not take too much time to simply explain that stress commonly causes this type of symptom and that effective treatment is available. If we are careful to avoid blaming the patient, validate that the symptoms are real and not imaginary, and offer to help, most patients will be able to accept this diagnosis. On their own, these steps can be therapeutic. You can then point them towards resources that offer education about PPD and self-guided treatment programs (see below and the appendix).

## Table 4.2: Summary of Educational, Cognitive and Behavioral Interventions

**Education about PPD**

Understand that the symptoms are real, but not caused by a structural abnormality

Recognize that symptoms are caused by neural pathways that have been learned and can be deactivated

Develop hope and the belief that they will recover

Personalize the information to help the patient see how this concept applies to them

**Cognitive and behavioral techniques**

Reduce fear in relation to symptoms

Take control over symptoms

Be more active and challenge triggers to symptoms

Practice outcome independence by paying less attention to symptoms while reengaging in activities

Practice mindful awareness of thoughts and feelings

Learn to identify emotions as they arise, especially when connected to symptom onset or exacerbation

Practice giving compassion to self and to oneself at earlier ages

Perform expressive writing exercises

Take action in life to stand up for oneself and create self-fulfillment

Practice meditative exercises to calm the brain

Work on forgiveness for self and others

Remind oneself that one is safe and not in danger

Engage more fully in life, work, exercise, play, and awe

Develop and maintain meaningful social connections

Define and act to create meaning and purpose

Busy clinicians will need to work with individual patients in a gradual way over time. Visits can focus on one or two brief interventions as described above, with follow-up appointments as needed. An initial visit of one hour, followed by three or four visits of 20-30 minutes each is sufficient for most patients to make the diagnosis of PPD, educate the patient, and initiate some of the behavioral interventions. A significant proportion of patients with psychophysiologic disorders will respond to these brief office interventions. While many clinicians may not have enough time or interest to perform the cognitive and behavioral interventions, they can make the diagnosis of PPD, explain what PPD is, and refer patients to mental health professionals who are experienced in dealing with psychophysiologic disorders. A critical message to give to patients at the end of each visit is that they are not damaged and that they can get better.

Many patients are motivated to work on these issues themselves. Resources containing self-guided PPD recovery programs are available (Schubiner and Betzold, 2016; Schubiner, 2016; Clarke, 2007; Hanscom, 2016; Oldfield, 2015; Schechter, 2014; Ozanich, 2012; Sachs, 2013; PPD Recovery Program at www.tmswiki.org). There are also a variety of additional interventions that can be helpful to reduce fear, increase confidence, and create contentment. Activities that help patients be active physically and socially are useful. Physical therapy can be important in recovery, especially if it is done to increase strength and flexibility and if the therapist avoids giving messages that the body is damaged. There are mindfulness meditation teachers in most major cities in the world. Exercise, yoga and Pilates classes are excellent adjuncts for many patients.

The following chapters consist of an introduction to the psychophysiology of emotions and a detailed description of therapeutic emotional interventions that can be used by trained medical or mental health providers to assist in the recovery of patients with PPD. They are often necessary in those individuals who fail to respond adequately to education, cognitive-behavioral strategies, and self-directed treatment modules. They can also be useful for those who choose to more fully face some of the emotionally charged issues in their lives.

## CHAPTER 4 SUMMARY

- *Once the patient accepts the diagnosis of PPD, you can begin treatment.*

- *The patient can be counseled to reduce the danger/alarm mechanism in the brain by calming the brain in the face of pain.*

- *Encourage increased physical and social activities without fear of harm.*

- *Facilitate self-compassion and forgiveness.*

- *Some patients may need to make changes in their lives to reduce stress.*

CHAPTER **5**

# Physiology and Psychology of Emotions

IN THIS CHAPTER, WE REVIEW HOW non-secure attachments in childhood and interruptions to secure attachments can produce a range of somatic signs and symptoms of PPD. We will also contrast these somatic signs and symptoms with features of healthy emotional experiencing. Hence, we will examine the physiology of emotions and some pathophysiological processes that interrupt healthy emotional experiencing. This aspect of PPD causation commonly needs to be focused on with patients not responding to the steps provided in chapters 2-4. This chapter provides a foundation for an emotion-focused assessment and treatment approach to PPD called Intensive Short-term Dynamic Psychotherapy (ISTDP). Much of this understanding was made possible by decades of videotape research in order to develop an in-depth understanding of emotions, anxiety, unconscious operations and healing operations of the mind (Davanloo, 2005; Abbass, 2015).

## Attachment

From the moment of our birth we are driven to attach to others. If you think of an image of a young baby and mother, face to face, smiling and moving in reaction to each other, it gives you a nice feeling. A healthy, secure attachment process is occurring and that infant is developing basic trust in people and indeed in the world: she is learning that she is loved and that the world is a safe place. She trusts that her parent will be affectionate, available and meet her emotional and developmental needs. Through these caring interactions over time she will also learn what her feelings are and how to express them adaptively. Through this optimal situation, her nervous system becomes set at a calm baseline level with ability to flexibly respond as needed to external stressors. If this bond continues without major ruptures she will grow up with the ability to know her own feelings, learn how to interact with others and to feel secure in herself. She will not have undue fear, anxiety or defensiveness. This is the fulfillment of the basic core human drive to attach to others as a foundation to mature and to successfully navigate the world (Bowlby, 1988).

## Attachment Trauma

But what happens if this securely attached child's bond is interrupted somehow, such as by mental illness in a parent, death of a parent, abuse, marital separation or any other adverse childhood event that disrupts that bond? This disruption results in fear and painful feelings related to this loss. If the child has other positive loving relationships to compensate for this trauma, she can process the feelings about this interrupted attachment and continue on a healthy developmental path. However, if the child does not have others who can help her experience these feelings she may begin to avoid both her own feelings and human relationships. Moreover, if the pain is very intense, as often occurs with trauma in the first few years of life, it will mobilize a reactive rage towards that person. The developing child will not be able to experience the rage on a conscious level and it will become buried. The child's unconscious mind will feel that she had actually acted out the rage toward the parent and a proportional amount of guilt will be fused with the rage.

This mixture of powerful guilt-laden unconscious feelings leads to anxiety, avoidance of all emotions, problems with closeness and intimacy and self-destructive behavior patterns. Her nervous system maybe stuck on alert, in constant unconscious fear of being harmed or doing harm. In this setting, she is likely to develop psychophysiological disorders in addition to conditions such as anxiety, depression, personality disorders, eating disorders and substance use disorders.

Trauma that is frequent, intense and occurs early in life creates more severe emotional pain, rage and guilt, which leads to a greater likelihood of severe disturbances. For example, if the attachment trauma is in infancy, the resultant unconscious anxiety will tend to manifest as cognitive-perceptual disruption resulting in a person with very poor anxiety tolerance, poor ability to maintain an integrated self and general difficulty navigating in the world (Davanloo, 2000; Abbass, 2015).

Likewise, if the parent-child attachment is insecure or disorganized to begin with, the child is vulnerable to similar severe disturbances due to the absence of a bond to assist in the development of self-reflective ability and anxiety tolerance among other healthy attributes (Schulte and Petermann, 2011). This situation of childhood neglect can thus lead to difficulties with self-caring, self-reflecting, tolerating anxiety and relating to others. Such individuals are commonly diagnosed with dissociative disorders or severe personality disorders in addition to PPDs.

## Figure 5.1: **Attachment and Attachment Trauma**

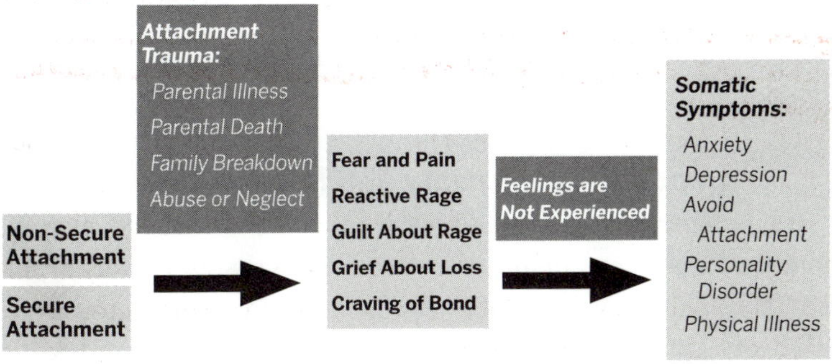

| Non-Secure Attachment / Secure Attachment | Attachment Trauma: Parental Illness, Parental Death, Family Breakdown, Abuse or Neglect | Fear and Pain, Reactive Rage, Guilt About Rage, Grief About Loss, Craving of Bond | Feelings are Not Experienced | Somatic Symptoms: Anxiety, Depression, Avoid Attachment, Personality Disorder, Physical Illness |

### Transference

The complex feelings related to attachment trauma are triggered in a patient's current relationships, especially in relation to healthcare professionals. Why? As a healthcare provider, you are a caring person, offering a potential attachment and expressing positive regard for your patient. You, looking into her eyes, remind her of her early attachments and the feelings about the ultimate fate of those attachments. This process of activating previously buried emotions and secondary anxiety and defenses in current relationships is called *transference* (see figure 5.2).

**Figure 5.2: Transference**

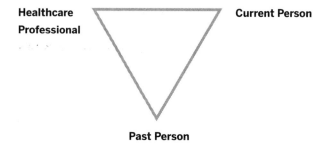

*Countertransference* refers to the identical process happening within the clinician. The possible attachment with the patient stirs a range of feelings in the professional. If the professional is aware of these feelings, he or she can use them as tools to understand and engage the patient in a helpful way. If the feelings are unprocessed, they can activate anxiety, depression, somatic symptoms or defenses resulting in harm to current relationships and to one's healthcare practice overall.

### Unconscious Anxiety and Related Defenses

When these unprocessed feelings are mobilized in your interview, patients manifest specific patterns of unconscious anxiety and defenses against this anxiety that you can detect, diagnose and work with (figure 5.3). In this section, we review the different patterns of unconscious anxiety and corresponding patterns of unconscious defense that typically occur.

## Figure 5.3: Triangle of Conflict

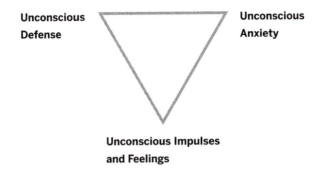

## Voluntary (Striated) Muscle Unconscious Anxiety

The first pattern is called *striated muscle anxiety*. While striated muscle is under voluntary control, it can also be activated by unconscious impulses and feelings. Striated muscle anxiety is a neurobiological process that starts in the thumbs and goes up to the hands, arms, shoulders, neck, and then it goes to the chest then the abdomen, legs and feet. It typically follows an orderly progression in the brain up the sensorimotor cortex. When it is activated, there are specific manifestations in the body that can be seen. The most obvious signs of this anxiety are hand clenching and sighing respirations as the muscles in the chest and diaphragm contract and relax.

A person with anxiety in this pathway on a chronic basis often has muscle spasms and musculoskeletal pain that can cause fibromyalgia, headache, backache, neck pain, shoulder pain, chest pain and abdominal wall pain. Other common signs of striated anxiety may include symptoms of a panic, including hyperventilation with dizziness, tingling in the hands and feet and a sense of shortness of breath. Furthermore, choking sensations, vocal problems, tics and tremors can be caused or worsened by unconscious anxiety in the relevant striated muscle (Abbass, 2005; Abbass, 2015).

**Table 5.1: Medical Presentations Caused and or Worsened by Striated Muscle Unconscious Anxiety**

| | | |
|---|---|---|
| Headache | Choking sensations | Neck pain |
| Chest Pain | (Globus) | Cramps |
| Jaw pain (TMJ) | Abdominal wall pain | Tremor |
| Shortness of breath | Vocal and other Tics | Back pain |
| Fibromyalgia | Leg pain | |

## Self-Reflection on Feeling States

When the person can self-reflect about his emotional states he can recognize that he has feelings of love, anger, guilt or grief. People who can identify the emotions may be mindful or self-reflective enough to use intellectual means of coping with their life stresses. However, if they are not able to actually feel the emotions, the anxiety may remain manifest as striated muscle tension perpetuating these somatic symptoms. Self-reflection and striated muscle tension are seen operating together: this is one explanation for why cognitive or intellectual insight into one's problems alone is often inadequate to reduce chronic pain in patients with fibromyalgia and related muscle-tension-linked conditions.

## Smooth Muscle Unconscious Anxiety

The second pathway of unconscious anxiety involves the *smooth muscle*. Smooth muscle is involuntary muscle under control of the autonomic nervous system. These include muscles in the airways, bowel, urinary bladder and blood vessels (see table 5.2). People with significant anxiety that activates these muscles suffer with a range of somatic symptoms leading to referral to medical specialists (Abbass 2005; Abbass, 2015).

## Repression

*Repression* is a deeply unconscious process where emotions are shunted away from consciousness. In other words, people with repressed emotions are unable to recognize or identify that these emotions are present. This process differs from *suppression* that consists of a conscious avoidance of emotions.

Repression is commonly seen with smooth muscle anxiety and cognitive-perceptual disruption (discussed below).

**Table 5.2: Medical Presentations Caused and or Worsened by Smooth Muscle Unconscious Anxiety**

| Medical Specialty | Smooth Muscle Related Condition |
|---|---|
| Cardiology | Hypertension, coronary spasm, Raynaud's phenomena, flushing, hypotension with loss of consciousness |
| Respiratory | Asthma, choking symptoms |
| Gastroenterology | Irritable Bowel Syndrome, Gastroesophageal Reflux Disease, functional vomiting, unexplained abdominal pain |
| Urology | Bladder dysfunction, Interstitial Cystitis |
| Neurology | Migraine |

## Cognitive-perceptual Disruption

*Cognitive-perceptual disruption* occurs when unconscious anxiety interrupts a person's special senses and ability to think. Some of the many manifestations of this anxiety include interruption of vision or hearing with what is better known as *sensory conversion*: a person can transiently go completely blind or deaf. The mind goes blank and the person can even lose consciousness with a fainting attack or a pseudoseizure type of event. The person can hallucinate when anxious: thus, he may actually experience transient psychotic phenomenon. These patients end up seeing the neurologist and having special tests like magnetic resonance imaging scans. A partial list of clinical presentations of cognitive-perceptual disruption is in table 5.3.

Patients with cognitive-perceptual disruption have poor memories and tend to be confused in the clinical setting. With a focus on his problems or his unconscious feelings, this patient will become increasingly confused or develop some other sensory phenomena as listed.

### Table 5.3: Cognitive-Perceptual Disruption Related to Medical Presentations

| | |
|---|---|
| Visual blurring, visual loss, | Loss of consciousness |
|    Tunnel vision | Pseudoseizure |
| Hearing impairment or loss | Dissociation |
| Memory loss, mental confusion | Hallucination in all five senses |

## Projection and Projective Identification

*Projection* is when one's own feelings and impulses are seen as being in another person. For example, a patient who is feeling angry inside becomes afraid you are going to strike him. *Projective identification* is when one thinks of another person as having attributes of themselves. A patient may think of you as being an ideal rescuer, a manipulative abuser, a neglecter, or a hateful critic. These projected parts may create a parallel or opposite reaction in the patient as they act in response to their perceptions of the professional.

Both projection and projective identification are commonly seen in association with cognitive-perceptual disruption. Many patients with dissociative and psychotic disorder diagnoses have both these manifestations of unconscious anxiety and defense operating at times.

## Motor Conversion

One other somatic pattern related to unconscious feelings is *motor conversion*. When this type of conversion is active, striated muscle groups become weak and lose power (as opposed to becoming tense as in striated muscle anxiety described above). For example, patients may lose ability to move their arms, legs or vocal cords.

When the person has motor conversion, they tend to look quite relaxed because they have low striated muscle tone. This is a well-known phenomenon observed with conversion called "la belle indifference" where the person appears relieved despite paralysis. Simply put, the patient is neither anxious nor defensive because the anxiety and defense are all manifesting as muscle weakness (Abbass, 2005; Abbass, 2015).

## Spectrum of Patients Suitable for Emotion Diagnostic Assessment

Following are categories of patients you will see with attachment trauma and problems with unconscious feelings and impulses who can benefit from emotion-based assessment and ISTDP. There are two spectra of patients (Davanloo, 2000; Abbass, 2015): the *spectrum of psychoneurotic disorders* which includes low, moderate and highly resistant patients and the *spectrum of patients with fragile character structure* (See Figure 5.4 and 5.5)

### The Low Resistant Patient

Low resistant patients only have unprocessed grief about losses. There is no anger, guilt, or self-criticism creating unconscious anxiety. In these patients, there is grief related to some loss of attachment figures in the past, usually after the age of eight. This grief is typically activated by recent relationship losses or with the start of a new relationship. These patients do not present with significant relational, somatic or psychiatric complaints. They do not experience smooth muscle anxiety or cognitive-perceptual disruption. Treatment is brief and consists of helping the patient feel grief about their losses (Abbass, 2015).

### The Moderate Resistant Patient

A moderate resistant patient has significant amounts of guilt-laden rage of murderous intensity, typically due to attachment trauma from age 5-7. There is a great deal of buried guilt about this rage. In addition, there is grief due to the early losses as well as from subsequent losses. All of these feelings and impulses are held in the unconscious by emotional detachment and habitual avoidant interpersonal defenses such as passivity or compliance. This unconscious anxiety is manifest as striated muscle tension that can result in muscle related symptoms and signs.

## Figure 5.4: **Spectra of Suitable Patients**

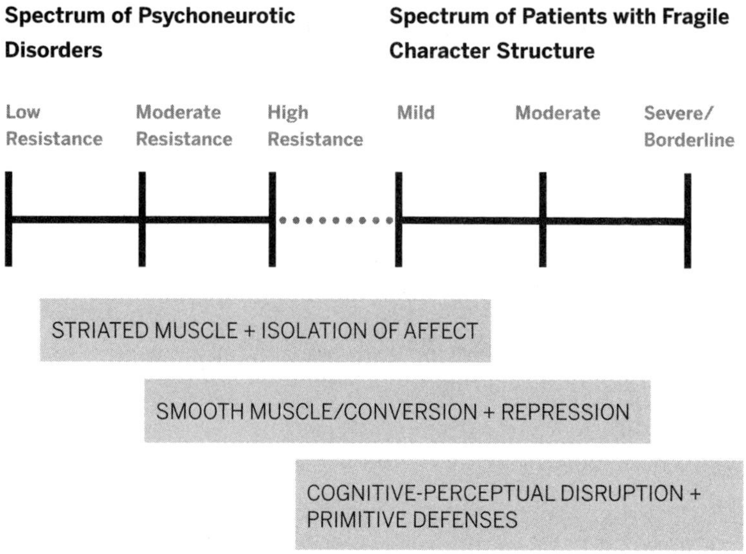

**Spectrum of Psychoneurotic Disorders**

**Spectrum of Patients with Fragile Character Structure**

| Low Resistance | Moderate Resistance | High Resistance | Mild | Moderate | Severe/ Borderline |
|---|---|---|---|---|---|

STRIATED MUSCLE + ISOLATION OF AFFECT

SMOOTH MUSCLE/CONVERSION + REPRESSION

COGNITIVE-PERCEPTUAL DISRUPTION + PRIMITIVE DEFENSES

## The Highly Resistant Patient

The highly resistant patient has multiple layers of unconscious rage and guilt. These correspond to different ages of trauma. Thus, the unconscious is organized into layers of increasingly intense rage coupled with guilt about the rage. There are also different layers of grief related to the significant losses and destructive effect of these losses. These patients are therefore typically highly defensive, emotionally detached, self-defeating and avoidant of genuine closeness. If one is not careful, it is easy to argue with, detach from or criticize these patients. They may present with abnormalities of smooth muscle and may have motor conversion and episodes of major depression.

## Fragile Character Structure

Patients with fragile character structure have intense unconscious feelings of primitive rage and guilt. There are layers of these emotions related to the key people in the past who have failed to consolidate a bond with them or who have abandoned or victimized them. There is also extensive craving of attachment and grief about failed attachment efforts. The major defenses are projective processes and repression so that they are generally unaware of these strong emotions. Poor impulse control, substance abuse, eating disorders and self-injury are common in this population. Unconscious anxiety is primarily manifest as cognitive-perceptual disruption.

Thus, it is often difficult to facilitate a healing process with these individuals because of the distorted perceptions the patient may form of their health professional and the strong feelings triggered in the care provider when working with these patients. When fragile character structure is detected, treatment referral to a mental health professional should be considered.

**Figure 5.5: Spectra of Patients and Feelings Impulses**

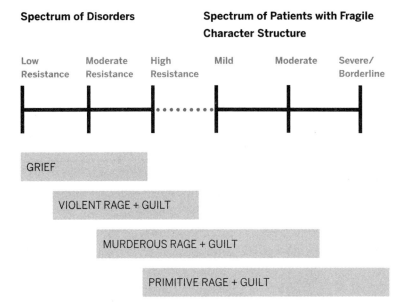

**Emotional Experiencing**

In contrast to the pathophysiological markers of unconscious unprocessed feelings and impulses described above, the actual experience of emotions is comprised of healthy physiologic events (Abbass, 2015).

### Positive Feelings

Positive feelings, including loving feelings are experienced typically with warmth in the chest or an upward moving energy. There is often an urge to reach out and embrace. People often smile and their bodies are relaxed as they experience calmness and lightness.

### Rage

When rage is actually experienced and felt, its somatic pathway begins from the bottom of the body in the feet or the lower abdomen and moves upward often with a heat or energy sensation, like a volcano. This sensation typically moves up toward the neck and towards the sides of the head and down the arms to the hands. Once the rage reaches the hands, there is typically an accompanying impulse to use the hands to grab and do some form of violence. If the rage has an urge to bite then the heat and energy are present in the muscles of the jaw. As this rage is experienced it displaces the unconscious anxiety in striated muscle. Thus, the person goes from tense and restrained to activated and free to move. Pain related to striated muscle tension is immediately reduced or removed when rage is felt.

### Guilt About Rage

The somatic experience of guilt consists of constriction of the upper chest and neck regions. When guilt is activated and experienced, people sob heavily and experience remorse about their rageful impulses as if they have just harmed loved ones. Guilt typically passes in distinct waves. When one is in the middle of a wave of significant guilt, it is difficult for the person to speak as they are in the grips of this intense emotion. When guilt is experienced it typically has a powerful effect of removing somatic symptoms that were being experienced in the session.

### Grief

In contrast to guilt, grief is not necessarily seen in distinct waves. However, tears of sadness and loss are present. There is rarely physical pain attached to the experience of grief.

Grief is also different from guilt in that the thoughts attached to grief relate to losses as opposed to remorse. Reductions of both striated and smooth muscle related symptoms occur when grief is experienced.

## CHAPTER 5 SUMMARY

- *Attachment trauma causes a range of complex emotions to be produced and buried.*

- *These complex feelings are mobilized in current relational situations including the professional-patient relationship.*

- *Unconscious anxiety and corresponding defenses are markers of unprocessed feelings and impulses.*

- *Healthy emotional experiencing has a specific physiology which is distinct from unconscious anxiety.*

CHAPTER **6**

# Psychodiagnostic Evaluation

USING THE UNDERSTANDING OF THE emotional operations described in chapter 5, you can examine unprocessed feelings and observe the direct effects of these emotions on physical symptoms toward ruling in or ruling out emotional factors as a cause of your patient's somatic problems (Abbass, 2015). Here we examine a step-by-step evaluation process.

**Figure 6.1: Psychodiagnosis**

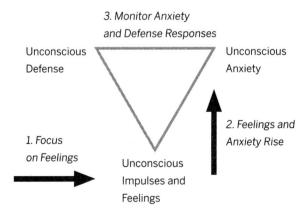

## Psychodiagnosis

### 1. Explain the Assessment Process to the Patient

By this point in the relationship with your patient, you will have established trust through listening to him, investigating his problems and offering your understanding of his problems. You will have established yourself as a caring knowledgeable person doing your best to assist him. These processes of relationship building are therapeutic on their own. They are also essential to go to the next step of exploring unconscious emotional processes.

First, explain to the patient that you and he are going to examine together whether or not emotions are linked to his somatic symptoms. Explain that you will ask about situations of stress or emotions to see if this focus changes the physical symptoms he is experiencing. Ask him to explore the process with you and to tell you what he notices as you speak together.

### 2. Focus to Activate Avoided Feelings

Begin by focusing on the situations and stressors that make the symptoms worse. Ask probing questions to identify which emotions your patient was feeling during those situations. This focus on specific situations and feelings will mobilize avoided unconscious feelings, unconscious anxiety and defenses against this anxiety (figure 5.1).

While focusing on emotions, observe any physical responses the patient may have. For example, you may note hand clenching, sighing respirations, you may hear stomach rumblings, or you might notice some degree of mental confusion. While conducting this interview, encourage the patient to notice phenomena together with you and clarify what you are observing to allow you and the patient a direct view of how emotions affect his body and behavior.

### 3. Differentiate Feelings, Anxiety, Defenses and Thoughts

One hallmark of psychophysiologic disorders is the inability to differentiate feelings in the body from anxiety, behaviors, defenses or thoughts. If a person can see the difference between these phenomena it will reduce symptoms and help him develop emotional mastery. It can also set the stage for him to begin to feel the feelings within his body leading to healing of wounds related to past attachment trauma.

### 4. Summarize Findings: Linking

To encourage self-reflection, summarize the findings as you focus on incidents with the patient. Short summaries can be used to tie together feelings, anxiety and defenses and the links between past and current relationship situations. This review helps the person learn to self-reflect and this alone can reduce symptoms and improve mastery over emotions (see chapter 4).

We will now review four cases to describe the psychodiagnostic evaluation of patients with the four common pathways.

### Case Vignette: Striated Muscle Tension

*A 54-year-old man diagnosed with fibromyalgia and chronic fatigue and was on disability from work. He is sitting with hands firmly clenched, his arms tense and his shoulders raised and tense while describing an incident of conflict with his wife.*

**Doctor (Dr):** So we now have a good idea about your symptoms and how they affect you. Can we look together now at how emotional stress affects your body to see if emotions make your symptoms worse? *[Clarifying task and gaining consent.]*

**Patient (Pt):** That sounds good.

**Dr:** OK. As we go let me know what you observe and I will point out what I see as well so we can figure this out together. *[Clarifying roles and partnership.]*

**Pt:** That sounds like a good way to go.

**Dr:** Can you describe a specific time when you had stressful event? *[Focus on specific incident.]*

**Pt:** Yes. Last week my wife and I got in a conflict over me talking to the lady who lives up the street.

**Dr:** What kind of conflict was it?

**Pt:** Um, well my wife's opinion was that I spent too much time talking to this lady and she was probably right.

**Dr:** So she brought this up in that incident?

**Pt:** Uh huh.

**Dr:** And how did you feel? *[Focus on feelings.]*

**Pt:** Well, I'm getting tired of hearing about this. *[Intellectual answer.]*

**Dr:** How do you feel towards her? *[Focus on feelings.]*

**Pt:** Mad. *[Deep sigh, clenching his hands.]*

**Dr:** Mad, like you mean angry?

**Pt:** Angry, yeah.

**Dr:** How do you experience the anger physically inside your body? *[Focus to experience the anger.]*

**Pt:** Physically?

**Dr:** Yeah. Physically how does it feel? *[Focus to experience the anger.]*

**Pt:** I'm very, very tense, and I get sore.

**Dr:** You get sore? *[Differentiating anger and anxiety/pain. Linking anger to pain.]*

**Pt:** Yeah, in my muscles, my shoulders. *[Hands strongly clenching.]*

**Dr:** So that's tension and anxiety. *[Differentiating anger from anxiety.]*

**Pt:** Anxiety, yeah.

**Dr:** But how did you experience the anger towards her? *[Focus to experience the anger.]*

**Pt:** It's hard to explain.

**Dr:** You became anxious and tense, did you? *[Linking anger to pain.]*

**Pt:** Yeah, I became anxious.

**Dr:** Do you become tense and sore when you have anger inside? *[Linking feelings to anxiety and pain.]*

**Pt:** Yeah and then I start to ignore her. *[Defense of avoidance.]*

**Dr:** That's a mechanism you use to deal with the anger and anxiety? But how do you experience the anger underneath? *[Differentiating defensive action versus feeling.]*

**Pt:** Like I say it's really hard to put a word on that. I get really mad, ok.

**Dr:** So it's like rage.

**Pt:** It's like rage, yeah.

**Dr:** How do you experience the rage physically? *[Focus to experience the anger.]*

**Pt:** *[Deep sigh.]*

This man was able to intellectually tell me how he felt towards his wife. He was able to identify the feeling, being "mad," on an intellectual basis. However, he was not actually feeling the rage, but rather the rage was resulting in striated muscle tension and muscular pain. This was evident by the clenched arms and hands and the sighing respirations and him noting the rise in pain. When the feelings toward his wife were activated his body froze up with tension. He did not recognize the rage nor did he experience or feel the rage, but when asked, can intellectually tell you he has rage. This awareness of feelings devoid of the experience of the feelings is an example of *intellectual self-reflection*, otherwise known as *isolation of affect*. When the person can intellectualize in this way, the anxiety manifests as striated muscle tension. Of the anxiety discharge pathways, this is the best one to have as it involves less repression of emotions and is generally easier to reverse. However, it is a pathway that was causing this man a great deal of muscle pain and the diagnosis of fibromyalgia. When he was assisted to experience the underlying rage, guilt and grief about his childhood trauma being triggered with his wife, he had a rapid and persistent resolution of the muscle tension and pain.

## Case Vignette: Smooth Muscle Unconscious Anxiety

*A middle-aged woman with migraine and irritable bowel syndrome is sitting looking very calm with no visible muscle tension.*

**Dr:** Can you tell me an example of when you had a conflict so we can see how it affects your symptoms? *[Clarifying task and focusing on a specific example.]*

**Pt:** If I ever get in a conflict with someone, I get a headache. *[Suggests link to complex feelings.]*

**Dr:** Can you describe a specific time this happened? *[Focus on specific incident.]*

**Pt:** It happens with my husband sometimes.

**Dr:** Can you tell me an example of when that happened? *[Focus on specific incident.]*

**Pt:** Yes, once when my husband had spent all our money on a trip and we had none left for our rent, I was so mad and I yelled at him. A while later I got a headache and felt nauseous.

**Dr:** So you did the action of yelling, but how did you feel toward him? *[Differentiating action versus feeling.]*

**Pt:** I thought "I'm not a good wife." *[Self-criticism. No signals of striated muscle anxiety.]*

**Dr:** You mean you became critical of yourself? *[Clarification of thought versus feelings.]*

**Pt:** Yes, I was. My stomach doesn't feel good right now.

**Dr:** Can you tell me what you notice in your stomach? *[Intellectual review to reduce anxiety and isolate affect.]*

**Pt:** There are cramps here, like bloating coming on. *[Points to her middle abdomen.]*

**Dr:** So when we talk about this situation of conflict and frustration, your stomach reacts. Is that what happened? *[Intellectually linking feelings of anger and anxiety with somatic symptoms.]*

**Pt:** Yes, it seems to.

**Dr:** So is this a way that frustration with your husband goes, to your stomach or to a headache somehow? Because when you start to talk about your frustration toward him, your stomach reacts here in the office and out there you got a headache. *[Repeat linking to increase self- reflection and reduce anxiety.]*

**Pt:** Yes, it did.

**Dr:** Can we examine how that happens here? *[Focus on task and her motivation and assent to proceed.]*

**Pt:** I would sure like to.

## Monitoring of Response

The doctor observes that this patient has no visible striated muscle tension. Her anxiety is not discharged into the striated muscle but is being repressed into the smooth muscle in the gastrointestinal tract. In the actual event she described, it appeared to produce headache. The patient also has a tendency to self-criticize when she has anger with someone else, another typical finding in patients with repression. To confirm that anxiety is channelling to the smooth muscle, and to ascertain the level of anxiety intolerance this patient has, the process is repeated with another focus.

**Dr:** Can you tell me what happens when we are here together? *[Focus to identify feelings.]*

**Pt:** Yes.

**Dr:** What feelings come up here with me as we talk together? *[Focus to identify feelings.]*

**Pt:** Well, I don't know. *[Smiling but no visible tension.]*

**Dr:** Let's see what feelings come up here that may generate this stomach effect? *[Repeat focus.]*

**Pt:** I... my stomach is reacting again. *[Patient looks totally relaxed with no striated muscle response.]*

**Dr:** So again, when you talk about your feelings, your stomach reacts with cramps. *[Recapitulation, linking feelings with anxiety.]*

**Pt:** Yes. I can see that now.

**Dr:** So there is a process that leads to your feelings being shut down and not directly felt in these situations. Instead your stomach reacts or you develop a headache. So the feelings seem to disappear this way. *[Recapitulation, linking feelings with anxiety.]*

**Pt**:   I see that now. I didn't really know that. My
stomach feels a bit better now. *[Hands clench and
she takes a sigh.]*

## Repression

Was this woman able to identify which emotions she was
feeling? No. She started to talk about a situation of irritation but
ended up talking about where the feelings went - into the stomach.
The emotions were *instantly repressed*. The feelings did not reach
consciousness but instead were repressed into the body.

## Anxiety Pathways

Thus, we confirmed that this woman's unconscious anxiety
was not discharged to the striated muscle but rather into the smooth
muscle of her bowel. She had limited ability to self-reflect on her
feelings. These findings show that rapid mobilization of unconscious
feelings could worsen her gastrointestinal symptoms because her
anxiety tolerance was not sufficient. Hence, before helping her to
be able to tolerate her feelings, you will need to first help her build
anxiety tolerance. As shown above when we intellectually reviewed
the links between her feelings and symptoms, the anxiety shifted to
the striated muscle (sighing respiration) and her stomach symptoms
reduced; encouraging self-reflection on affect caused the anxiety
to go away from repression and into striated muscle, temporarily
relieving her stomach symptoms.

## Evaluation and Planning: Smooth Muscle

This symptom activation when focusing on feelings
and symptom reduction with intellectual review is important
diagnostic data pointing to an emotional cause of her symptoms.
Through this evaluation we also see she will need help to build
more anxiety tolerance to enable her to identify and feel her own
emotions rather than developing symptoms. We will review a
treatment approach to this called the *graded format of ISTDP*,
in chapter 8 (Davanloo, 1990a; Whittemore, 1996; Abbass and
Bechard, 2007; Abbass, 2015).

### Case Vignette: Cognitive-Perceptual Disruption

*This is from a 13ᵗʰ treatment session with a 34-year-old man with paranoid personality disorder, episodes of mental confusion, and depression. He arrived in the session rubbing his eyes but with absolutely no striated muscle anxiety, such as hand clenching or sighing. In this segment you will see a means of symptom removal after reducing anxiety by reviewing the somatic symptoms and focusing on underlying causes.*

**Pt:** You'll have to excuse me today; I'm a little foggy headed.

**Dr:** Foggy? *[Clarification of the experience.]*

**Pt:** Yeah.

**Dr:** Is your thinking kind of foggy, cloudy? *[Clarification of the experience.]*

**Pt:** Foggy and cloudy, yeah.

**Dr:** How's your vision? *[Clarification of the experience.]*

**Pt:** Cloudy.

**Dr:** Do you have tunnel vision, or is it like looking through a screen? *[Clarification of the experience.]*

**Pt:** More tunnel vision.

**Dr:** More like it's hard to see the outside of your visual field, but you can see straight ahead in the room. *[Clarification of the experience.]*

**Pt:** Yeah.

**Dr:** When did that start?

**Pt:** Um, two, maybe two days ago relatively... like I just noticed it this morning.

**Dr:** So this is what we looked at as anxiety, right? *[Reminding him of previously learned material.]*

**Pt:** Yeah.

**Dr:** And the last two days, all day? *[Clarification of the experience.]*

**Pt:** Actually more or less just today when I woke up.

**Dr:** Okay, so why are you anxious right now? *[Focus to identify causes.]*

**Pt:** Is it anxiety?

**Dr:** That's what we figured when we've met before. *[Reminding him of previously learned material.]*

**Pt:** It's more of a completely drugged type of feeling.

**Dr:** It's a disconnection kind of thing. Disconnected from what's going on. *[Clarification.]*

**Pt:** Yeah.

**Dr:** And any thoughts about why you're anxious this morning? *[Focus to identify causes.]*

**Pt:** I don't think it has anything to do with coming here.

**Dr:** You don't think it has anything to do with coming in? *[Focus to identify causes.]*

**Pt:** Not to do with coming to see you, no.

**Dr:** You weren't anxious about it? *[Focus to identify causes.]*

**Pt:** No, I don't think so.

**Dr:** So how do we account for that anxiety then? How are you accounting for it? *[Focus to identify causes.]*

**Pt:** I've got work tomorrow and I was thinking about work last night.

**Dr:** Why today though? *[Focus to identify causes.]*

**Pt:** Um, I don't know. You're right, because it's kind of subsiding! *[Draws a large sigh.]*

**Dr:** It's just reduced now?

**Pt:** Yeah.

As with the last patient, there is no striated muscle anxiety signal at first. He was completely unaware of his anxiety and the underlying feelings. He wasn't even conscious that he was experiencing anxiety. Rather anxiety was manifest as cognitive and visual abnormalities. This is why these processes are called *unconscious* anxiety pathways. The lack of insight into the causes of the symptoms leads patients to emergency departments and doctor's offices rather than to a psychologist's office due to this lack of insight. By helping self-reflect on his body responses, the anxiety shifted to striated muscle (as evidenced by the sigh) reducing his visual symptoms.

## Projection and Projective Identification

In the early sessions with this patient, he was afraid of angry reactions from others. He was, thus, *projecting* hostility out on the world and interacting with it. By this point in therapy depicted above, he had largely ceased projecting and rather was allowing himself to examine his own emotions and be anxious about the emotions. In beginning to trust, his anxiety was beginning to manifest in cognitive-perceptual disruption. Projection and related primitive defenses, such as splitting into all good or all bad, are commonly seen in patients with cognitive-perceptual disruption: the two of these phenomena are seen in the same patients. As described, patients with this set of patterns typically have had non-secure attachments and major trauma.

## Motor Conversion

Another somatic pattern related to unconscious impulses and feelings is motor conversion. When motor conversion is active, instead of striated muscle tensing up, the patient goes weak and flat, losing power in one or more muscle groups. For example, the patient may lose the ability to move his arms, legs, or vocal cords. When the patient's anxiety goes into conversion, he looks relaxed because he has no striated muscle tone.

To clarify, many neurologists also refer to striated muscle unconscious anxiety symptoms (such as muscle spasms, excess muscle tension) as conversion, but the mechanism is different. Patients with anxiety in the striated muscle rarely show "la belle indifference;" patients with motor conversion usually do. Patients with anxiety in the striated muscle will show signalling of a rise of unconscious feeling and anxiety; patients with motor conversion do not. Patients with anxiety in the striated muscle will be tense and strong; patients with motor conversion will show no tension and lots of weakness. Patients with anxiety in the striated muscle will use various defenses including intellectualization; patients with motor conversion will show few defenses since all the feelings and anxiety are repressed, manifesting as weakness. Hence, the treatment of these two categories of conversion will differ greatly.

### Case Vignette: Motor Conversion

*A man with episodic weakness with falling and becoming at times paralyzed for hours or days comes to the office by wheelchair. He is very weak and moving from side to side in the chair as if he could fall out.*

> **Dr:** I understand you saw the neurologist about some problems and he suggested that we meet. What are the difficulties that you're experiencing at this point in time? [*Focus to specifics.*]
>
> **Pt:** [*Both arms and body listing to the right.*]
>
> **Dr:** You're experiencing physical symptoms right now? [*Clarification of symptoms, encouraging self-reflection.*]
>
> **Pt:** Yes.
>
> **Dr:** What are you experiencing in your body at this point, right now? What is it that you observe from inside? [*Encouraging self-reflection.*]
>
> **Pt:** Uh, well, I'm coherent. [*He is self-reflecting and his head is clear.*]
>
> **Dr:** Um-hmm, what is it that you're noticing in your body? [*Encouraging self-reflection.*]
>
> **Pt:** Okay. [*Self-reflecting.*]
>
> **Dr:** Are you aware of being anxious? [*Encouraging self-reflection.*]
>
> **Pt:** No, I'm not anxious.
>
> **Dr:** Do you notice any muscle tension? [*Encouraging self-reflection.*]

**Pt:** You mean as far as being nervous coming into the building?

**Dr:** Muscle tension within your body. *[Encouraging self-reflection.]*

**Pt:** Oh, yeah, I know that's there.

**Dr:** Why is that there right now when you're coming here to see me? What's causing that? What feelings are driving that tension in the body? *[Focus to identify feelings.]*

### Response to Focused Process

This patient had no sighing and hand clenching, suggesting the emotional forces are manifesting as conversion. After seven minutes of focusing on the bodily experiences and what underlying emotions he had, the patient became much more relaxed and the spasms stopped. He began to focus on conflict with his new wife that predated these symptoms by two years.

**Pt:** My wife likes to have things a certain way, and sometimes she goes off yelling and cursing.

**Dr:** Um-hmm.

**Pt:** And it really pisses me off.

**Dr:** So this was a certain time when you were home and that happened? *[Focus to specifics.]*

**Pt:** I could hear her walking around the hallway swearing.

**Dr:** So how do you feel toward her? *[Focus to identify feelings.]*

**Pt:** Very angry!

**Dr:** How does that feel in your body when you think about that — in your body? *[Focus to experience anger.]*

**Pt:** In my body. *[Self-reflecting.]*

**Dr:** Thinking about it now what are you noticing that tells you that you feel very angry inside? *[Focus to experience anger.]*

**Pt:**   Gosh! *[Self-reflecting, drawing a large sigh and hands are clenching.]*

## Moving Anxiety into Striated Muscle

This patient's sigh is a marker of a shift from motor conversion to the striated muscle anxiety pathway. This transition is a direct product of focus to mobilize his unconscious feelings coupled with efforts for him to observe his body and feelings. When he started to self-reflect, the emotional forces shifted from conversion to striated muscle anxiety. From this state he went on to experience some complex feelings about his wife, including a small amount of somatic anger and guilt. These feelings with his wife became linked to complex feelings about his mother from past verbal abuse. As he described the mother he felt strong anger in his body and also felt guilty about this anger. His mother is now a nice, older woman; the conflict with his wife had mobilized this unresolved rage and guilt from his childhood.

At the end of the session, the patient was quite strong in all his limbs and walked out with no need for his cane or wheelchair. What took place is the process of replacing motor conversion with emotional awareness and experience. We explored feelings gradually to change from motor conversion to the striated muscle anxiety. Chapter 8 describes this "graded format" in some detail, but the principle is this: if the therapist helps the patient reflect on his emotions and body responses, this causes unconscious anxiety to shift to the striated muscle away from other anxiety pathways.

## Interruption of Defensive Behavior

In the same way, some patients will tense up and guard during an abdominal examination, some patients will become more emotionally detached or defensive when you try to examine his emotional functions. The patient will begin to avoid both you and the experience of his feelings.

To handle this resistance, specific types of interventions are helpful. These interventions are on a spectrum from *focusing away from the defense* to *clarifying the defense* to *challenging the defense.* These steps are used with increasing intensity depending on how strongly the defense is working at that moment in the interview.

Focusing away from defense is encouragement to do the opposite thing the defense wants the patient to do. This is a first step to use when you encounter a defending patient. If the patient is only moderately resistant, as in the case illustrated in this chapter, this type of interventions is all you will need.

If the person defends more despite focusing way from the defense, then you will need to clarify or point out the defense. This pointing out will educate the patient about what he is doing and its impact on his own shared treatment goals. This intervention is needed with more moderately resistant and highly resistant patients who hold onto their defenses and resist giving them up. The striated muscle case in this chapter required a few such clarifications.

If the patient continues to defend despite clarification then challenge to the defense is required. Challenge is reserved for when you have adequately clarified the defenses and the patient understands the defense despite continuing to employ it. Hence, challenge to a defense is always done *in concert with the patient.* This will prevent any interruptions of your treating relationship. See table 6.1 for some examples of defenses and these levels of intervention.

This interruption of defense causes a rise in both unconscious feelings and anxiety that the defenses were covering. So when you clarify or challenge defenses, you will see signs of unconscious anxiety allowing you to diagnose PPD in many cases (see figure 6.1). The following vignette illustrates the evaluation process with a person who is highly intellectual and doesn't allow feelings to be felt.

### Case Vignette: Handling Defensive Behavior

*A 25-year-old man with chronic headaches presents in a very detached fashion with arms closed, avoiding eye contact. When we focused on his feelings, anxiety was generated and he became tense, more detached and intellectualized about his problems.*

*The headache stayed the same during this part of the interview. It became clear that for us to understand his emotional patterns, he would have to allow himself to actually feel some of his feelings in order to see the impact of feeling versus just thinking about feelings.*

### Table 6.1: Examples of Defenses and Ways to Handle Defenses

| Defense | Focus away from the defense | Clarify the defense | Challenge the defense |
|---|---|---|---|
| Passivity | Can we look into this together? | Do you notice you are waiting for me? | If you don't go passive. |
| Defiance | Do you want us to explore that? | It seems you are fighting yourself. | If you don't fight yourself. |
| Compliance | What would you like us to focus on? | Are you going along with me? | If you are not just going along with me. |
| Detachment | Can you stay present here with me? | Do you notice you avoid my eyes? | If you don't detach. |
| Intellectualization Rumination | How do you feel? | Do you notice you are thinking but not feeling? | If you don't think. |
| Self attack | We are here to do a good thing for you | Do you notice you beat yourself up? | If you don't attack yourself. |

*He is now sitting with his hands firmly clenched and taking frequent sighs. His anxiety is in striated muscle. He is intellectually ruminating about feelings. Thus, striated muscle anxiety could be causing or contributing to his chronic headache. To find out if this anxiety is a factor in his headache, we need to help him feel the feelings that he is tense about in the office. When he feels the feelings, the anxiety will drop and we will see the impact of this on his headache.*

**Dr:** We have figured this thing out intellectually, but we have to do something else. I think that to really see if feelings are causing part of your headaches, we're going to have to do something different than what we've done so far.

**Pt:** *[Nods head in agreement.]*

**Dr:** Because one thing is that you think a lot and analyse things. You go over things a lot in your thoughts, but I think that's causing you to cut off your feelings. The feelings are in one place in the brain and thoughts are in another place. *[Clarifying feelings versus intellectualization.]*

**Pt:** Mm hmm.

**Dr:** Can you hold off from thinking for a few minutes and see how you feel? *[Focusing away from defense.]* Can you not let yourself analyse for a minute and see what feelings you have that just show up and make you tense up? Would that be very hard to do? *[Clarifying defense.]*

**Pt:** Well, I'm used to always thinking about things. Like I can think about things all day long and worry a lot.

**Dr:** Constantly you're thinking? *[Clarifying defense.]*

**Pt:** Always.

**Dr:** To do that here though is going to interrupt your goal of seeing if blocked feelings are part of your problem though, right? *[Clarifying the defense.]*

**Pt:** Right. I don't know how to shut my thinking off.

**Dr:** But how can we do that? *[Encouragement to give up defense.]*

**Pt:** I don't know. *[Shakes head in helpless gesture.]*

**Dr:** But isn't that kind of a helpless thought if you think you can't do it? *[Clarifying defense of helplessness.]* See if you don't let yourself think helpless for a minute, how do you feel? *[Challenge to defense and focus on feelings.]* Don't let yourself doubt yourself for a minute. *[Challenge to defense.]* Just see how you feel there. *[Focus on feelings.]*

**Pt:** I know, I'm trying.

**Dr:** You have to not think though. *[Challenge to defense.]*

**Pt:** I see that.

**Dr:** See, there are several things you have to not do to let yourself feel something. *[Clarifying.]*

**Pt:** *[Still thinking to himself.]*

**Dr:** See you're thinking still. *[Clarifying defense.]*

**Pt:** I don't know how...

**Dr:** There's this thinking still happening, right? *[Clarifying defense.]*

**Pt:** Yes, I know. *[Takes a sigh signalling rise in feelings.]*

### Going in the Right Direction

This sighing and him acknowledging the defense means the defense is being weakened. Now the feelings and anxiety may rise allowing you to diagnose or rule out PPD. Since he now sees the defense but is still using it, you can use stronger interventions of challenge: this will help the feelings rise to a higher level and be experienced.

**Dr:** How do you feel underneath that if you don't let yourself think? *[Focus on feelings and challenge to defense.]* If you just hold off the thinking for a minute. *[Challenge.]*

**Pt:** I don't know, I don't know. I'm trying not to think and it's just happening.

**Dr:** So let's see how you feel underneath that. *[Focus on feelings.]*

**Pt:** Um. *[Breaks eye contact and detaching from doctor.]*

**Dr:** You have to not detach from me too because that would be another thing that would block your goal. *[Clarifying defense.]*

**Pt:** Right. *[Still detaching, avoiding eye contact.]*

**Dr:** You would have to not withdraw yourself or detach. See, you're withdrawing. *[Clarifying defense.]* How do you feel if you don't detach or withdraw or don't let a wall or barrier come up here? *[Focus on feelings and challenge to defense]*. How do you feel? *[Focus on feelings.]*

## Match Your Activity With the Level of Defenses

Notice here that I repeat the question about feelings, the clarification of defenses and challenge to defenses that arise. As long as the defenses are in operation, we must keep helping him both activate his feelings and interrupt his own defenses. Failing this we could not determine whether emotions are part of his somatic problems: he would just stay tense, detached and ruminating with a headache.

**Pt:** I feel kind of, I can't think of the word. That's what I'm actually trying to think of. *[Hands clenching, wringing.]*

**Dr:** You're gripping. You notice how tight you're gripping your hands? *[Pointing out anxiety.]*

**Pt:** Yeah, I know.

**Dr:** It's really tight.

**Pt:** I know.

**Dr:** But how do you feel if you don't do that to you? If you don't shut yourself down. *[Focus on feelings and challenge to emotional avoidance.]*

**Pt:** Okay, to tell you the truth I didn't want to come here. I don't know what that feeling is. I know I'm feeling something. I can't think of the word right now. *[Hands move freely, signalling drop in tension as he expresses frustration.]*

**Dr:** In your body?

**Pt:** Yes.

**Dr:** What do you feel in your body? What do you notice? *[Continued focus on feelings.]*

**Pt:**  Yes, I feel like I'm here because I have headaches.
I shouldn't be here talking about what feelings I feel.
I don't understand why I should be talking about
that. *[Referring to being frustrated at being sent for
emotion-based assessment.]*

**Dr:**  Mm hmm.

**Pt:**  I understand that it has something to do with
stress. And I know I block feelings but... *[He himself
explains what is so important about what we are
focusing on.]*

**Dr:**  But see, only if you want to. If you want us together
to see what's going on. *[Undoing any defiance and
ensuring that he wants to focus together.]* Obviously,
you're a very bright person and this is happening to
you.

**Pt:**  Right.

**Dr:**  And you're stuck with this tension happening to
you.

**Pt:**  Right.

**Dr:**  Rather than getting to feel your feelings you're
stuck with this. But, if you want us to, we can see what
drives that. *[Clarifying his will.]*

**Pt:**  I do want to.

**Dr:**  So how do you feel here with me, under this
muscle tension, if you don't let it go gripping, if you
don't let yourself detach and if you don't let yourself
think. *[Focus on feelings with challenge to defenses.]*
Let's just see how do you feel underneath that. *[Focus
on feelings.]*

**Pt:**  I actually kind of feel sad that I have to be in this
kind of place. No, that's not it. *[He is still intellectualizing
and ruminating but catches himself and interrupts it.]*

**Dr:**  Is that more of a thought?

**Pt:**  Yes. As soon as I found out I had to come here
when the doctor told me to come.

**Dr:** How did you feel towards your doctor when he referred you to me? *[Focus on feelings.]*

**Pt:** I felt anger because... *[Intellectual response.]*

**Dr:** How does that anger feel? When you were in his office you felt anger inside yourself towards him? *[Focus on feelings.]*

**Pt:** Yes.

**Dr:** How do you feel anger towards him in your body? *[Focus on feelings.]*

**Pt:** See I know I'm feeling anger but I just don't know how to feel that. *[Tension has dropped, hands moving in an expressive fashion. He is in contact with the experience of the anger.]*

**Dr:** How do you know you feel anger right there? What do you notice in your arms? *[Focus on feelings.]*

**Pt:** I'm not gripping anymore! *[He detects the drop in tension.]*

**Dr:** What have you got there instead? What do you notice? *[Focus on feelings.]*

**Pt:** I'm not tense anymore. My shoulders are relaxed.

**Pt:** Okay, so what changed that helped you know there is anger inside you there? The tension left? Is that what happened?

**Pt:** Yes.

**Dr:** What took its place for a second?

**Pt:** It was so fast. *[The feeling of anger.]*

**Dr:** Something fast?

**Pt:** Yes. It went right up my body. *[Somatic pathway of anger.]*

**Dr:** Something moved there?

**Pt:** Mm hmm. See, what I think happens is I do feel feelings but it's just so quick into the tension that I can't identify what they are. *[He summarizes how the anxiety and defenses block his feelings.]*

**Dr:** How is your forehead right now?

**Pt:** It's okay. It's better than it was. *[Frontal head pain reduction.]*

**Dr:** How about the top of your head?

**Pt:** That feels alright right now too. Yeah.

**Dr:** Alright. So did that pain all leave when the tension in your shoulders dropped?

**Pt:** Yeah.

In this vignette, we helped him to feel some of the feelings he was having that were creating striated anxiety and pain in his body. When he felt some feelings, his tension dropped and the pain dropped at the same time, confirming that the two were linked. Tension was a contributor to his pain: if he is able to feel his feelings the headaches should be reduced. In his case we had to help him interrupt his habitual avoidance of feelings to see that his symptoms were partly driven by striated muscle anxiety.

## Monitoring Somatic Pathways of Emotions

When the patient is able to identify or experience emotions, there are specific physical manifestations that can be seen in the interview. It is important to note the physical effects at the times when the patient is feeling emotions, such as grief over losses or guilt-laden anger over hurtful events to determine any linkage to somatic symptoms. The vignettes below demonstrate some details of the somatic pathways of emotions as observed in assessment interviews.

## Guilt, Somatic Symptoms, and Self-Directed Anger

Striated muscle anxiety, smooth muscle anxiety, cognitive-perceptual disruption, conversion and other symptoms are direct products of complex feelings including positive feelings, violent rage and guilt about the rage all toward the same person. Other manifestations of self-directed rage may include self-criticism, depression and defenses like passivity or helplessness. Thus, patients may develop somatic sensations or simply verbally state that they are angry at themselves.

Often a person will self-attack in this way when they are close to experiencing the feelings of rage and guilt. Pay close attention to the impact the self-attacking has on the patient's symptoms. By pointing out self-attacking, the clinician is helping the patient recognize that these symptoms are manifestations of anger directing inward: in some cases, symptoms will reduce simply with awareness of this process. In other cases, experiencing the anger and guilt is required for symptom removal.

### Case Vignette: Guilt And Symptom Reduction

*This sixty-year-old man with multiple medically unexplained symptoms arrived frustrated that the doctor was late for the appointment. When we focused on how he felt the anger inside his body, he developed abdominal pain. This confirmed that when anger is activated, it causes abdominal pain. When I clarified why the anger turned toward himself he said it was a lifelong pattern of avoiding aggression. We then focused on why he was so afraid of the feeling of anger and what he was afraid the anger would do if he hadn't directed it inward to his stomach.*

**Dr:** Let me ask you about the anger another way. If an uncivilized guy came in and has that anger in him what would he do? *[Focus on the impulse of his anger that he avoided.]*

**Pt:** I see him walking away. *[Avoidant pattern.]*

**Dr:** No, but if the guy comes at me. *[Focus on his impulse.]*

**Pt:** He doesn't confront you. He just turns and walks away. *[Avoidant pattern.]*

**Dr:** Let's turn him around to come at me so we can see the anger you're afraid of.

**Pt:**  You know what I see in my head, I see him standing up to you and saying, "I took the time to be here, so why couldn't you be on time?"

**Dr:**  So that is the civilized guy. What are you so afraid of when you have this anger in your body? *[Encouragement to see and experience the aggressive impulse.]*

**Pt:**  I don't know any other way to be. *[Arms move freely in expressive fashion.]*

**Dr:**  No? You've never seen aggression?

**Pt:**  Yes I have, but it upsets me terribly.

**Dr:**  Can you tell me?

**Pt:**  I went to see a boxing match with my neighbor one time and I cried about it for two days. It upset me to see men hitting each other.

**Dr:**  Put it this way; if a boxer comes in and has that anger in his body, and he comes over to me how much punching does he have inside of him if he let it out on me? *[Encouragement to see and experience the aggressive impulse.]*

**Pt:**  Just once because it's not a really big deal.

**Dr:**  One punch?

**Pt:**  One punch.

**Dr:**  Where does that go?

**Pt:**  Right in your face! *[Right fist clenched and punches into other hand, says with a smile.]*

**Dr:**  Let's take a look at it for a second. One shot in the face.

**Pt:**  Oh man, I'm really getting upset. *[Weeping and obviously feeling guilt.]*

**Dr:**  How would you feel if you had pounded on me a minute ago?

**Pt:**  Guilt. It would take me days to get over something like that. When my father does something absolutely stupid and I feel mad at him I get so guilty.

**Dr:**  Can you tell me one of those times?

**Pt:** I just noticed now that my stomach has stopped hurting.

**Dr:** Your stomach doesn't hurt now? What do you make of that?

**Pt:** Hmm.

**Dr:** It's as if your stomach absorbed the anger that was triggered. As if you actually would hurt me so you stuffed the anger in your stomach. Is that what happened? *[Recap linking feelings to anxiety and symptoms.]*

**Pt:** It must be that way. It just happened that way. *[Looks surprised.]*

**Dr:** But what we see is you have a lot of guilt about anger inside you because of good feelings? Then it's as if you had done harm with the anger and hurt someone you didn't want to hurt. *[More linking of avoided feelings to symptoms.]*

**Pt:** Yes, I see that.

**Dr:** And then you started to talk about your father and how that same pattern is there with him. Is this an old pattern of handling guilt about anger? *[More recapping.]*

**Pt:** I've been doing this since I was a kid. I could never stand up to my father.

This process helps the patient identify, feel and talk about his anxiety laden feelings triggered by me being late. These feelings included anger and guilt, as if he had hurt me. Obviously, these feelings were linked to the mixed feelings he had towards his father that he had not processed. When he was able to recognize and feel these mixed feelings it caused the anxiety in his body to stop and the stomach pain to cease. Prior to this, whenever anger was triggered it was repressed into his stomach creating pain. By helping him see and feel these mixed feelings, we helped him to see that avoided anger and guilt about anger are linked to his pain. At the same time, we have helped reduce his symptoms.

When he felt the feelings, his mind automatically linked these complex feelings to those of his father. This process is called *partial unlocking of the unconscious* (Davanloo, 1990b) and is examined in detail with case vignettes in *Reaching Through Resistance* (Abbass, 2015). The act of linking the complex feelings to the past brings both diagnostic insight and symptom reduction in most patients.

## Anxiety Reduction

As described, the interviewing process encourages the patient to identify and experience emotions. As this occurs, anxiety is activated, leading to a variety of somatic responses and defensive behaviors. If the anxiety rises too high and the patient is too uncomfortable or unable to think clearly, it is necessary to reduce the anxiety temporarily.

**Table 6.2: Techniques to Reduce Anxiety**

| Anxiety Reducing Technique | Example |
| --- | --- |
| Intellectual review of the bodily symptoms | Can you tell me how you are experiencing the anxiety in your body, in your hands, chest etc.? |
| Recapitulation and review of the information that has been learned: summarizing findings | So far, we see that when you have strong anger it triggers anxiety in the form of tension in your chest and shortness of breath. |
| Changing the topic from one area of focus to another: for example, going from one situation to another | Can you tell me about another example where this happened? |
| Focus on the feelings towards you at the time of interview | What feelings are coming up here with me and generating this anxiety as we talk? |
| Focus on guilt about any anger | How would you feel if that anger had come out and hurt your husband? |

There are several specific techniques to reduce anxiety (see table 6.1). One key method to reduce anxiety is to intellectualize about the process taking place in the office. Another is self-reflection about the body sensations: this is an example of a mindfulness type of intervention (see chapter 4) to help the patient use the self-observing centers of the brain to override excess stimulation from the emotional centers.

While reducing this anxiety, carefully observe the patient's responses to gather more diagnostic information on the relationship between anxiety and physical symptoms.

### Case Vignette: Anxiety Reduction

*This thirty-two-year-old man presented with severe anxiety interrupting his ability to think. He has no sign of striated muscle anxiety and looks somewhat confused. This observation suggests that his anxiety is manifesting as cognitive-perceptual disruption. This high anxiety requires techniques to reduce anxiety so the interview is tolerable and so that any links between anxiety and somatic symptoms can be made clear.*

**Dr:** I notice you are anxious.

**Pt:** Well it's sort of an ongoing thing more or less.

**Dr:** Ongoing anxiety?

**Pt:** Yeah.

**Dr:** What is it like physically when you experience it right now? How do you notice it? *[Focus on body cues to increase self-reflection.]*

**Pt:** Well um, well I have almost, for years, I get sick, I get dizziness. *[Speech is not fluent due to cognitive disruption.]*

**Dr:** Do you feel dizzy right now? *[Focus on body cues to increase self-reflection.]*

**Pt:** Yeah, dizziness. It goes from sort of a mild dizziness which is constant to dizzy spells like not spinning around but just sort of... they don't last very long but they're dizzy spells.

**Dr:** Right now when you have dizziness, is it that you're having a spinning sensation or just a feeling of being unstable? *[Focus on body cues to increase self-reflection.]*

**Pt:** More, more unstable.

**Dr:** Unstable sort of feeling like you're going to fall over you mean? *[Focus on body cues to increase self-reflection.]*

**Pt:** Yeah, I would have to hold on to something.

**Dr:** Do you feel unsteady even sitting down?

**Pt:** No, I'm okay, I'm pretty well okay now.

**Dr:** But do you feel unstable on your feet right now?

**Pt:** Yeah, *[nods head]* it's sort of that is associated with, I feel, not closed in but, like I can't keep track of the things around me.

**Dr:** Mm hmm.

**Pt:** There's too much information. Sort of like a tunnel type of vision. *[Perceptual disruption.]*

**Dr:** Your vision has tunnels, like looking through a tube? *[Focus on body cues to increase self-reflection.]*

**Pt:** Yeah, I can't take in too much information. *[Cognitive disruption.]*

**Dr:** I see. Is there anything else physically that you notice? Do you have sweating? *[Focus on other body cues to reduce anxiety by increasing self-reflection.]*

**Pt:** Yeah, well I have sweating, hot flashes.

**Dr:** Hot flashes. Do you have that right now? *[Focus on other body cues to reduce anxiety by increasing self-reflection.]*

**Pt:** No I don't have that right now. They're very bad though. I get like I'm in an oven or something.
Um and I have, I've never been able to explain it before but it feels like lightning shocks in my head.

**Dr:** Shock sensations in your head?

**Pt:** Yeah sort of bolts like lightning sometimes. It's a funny feeling. I can't explain it. *[Sigh and hands clenching: anxiety is converting to striated muscle.]*

**Dr:** Like zaps sort of. Do you have dry mouth and things like that right now? *[Focus on other body cues.]*

**Pt:** Yes.

**Dr:** Any sensations in your stomach that you have right now? *[Focus on other body cues.]*

**Pt:** Well my stomach is not too bad now but what happens to me when I have an anxiety period is it's always started by some sort of physical manifestation and it's almost always stomach cramps and diarrhea. *[Refers to smooth muscle anxiety.]*

**Dr:** Mm hmm.

**Pt:** And just a feeling of sickness like a poison in my body.

**Dr:** Feels miserable; a poisonous feeling inside your body, your stomach. *[Reflecting his experience of being poisoned by his anxiety.]*

**Pt:** Yes, in my stomach.

**Dr:** Mm hmm. So, in your stomach you might get diarrhea or cramps or some other kind of sensation.

**Pt:** Oh yeah.

**Dr:** Do you have anything else right now like a tingling in your hands and feet or any sensation in your arms? *[Focus on other body cues.]*

**Pt:** No, I don't have any of that. *[Sighs and hands clenching: striated muscle anxiety.]*

**Dr:** Mm hmm. And uh, how is your vision right now? Has it changed any since you came in?

**Pt:** Yeah, it's a little better, a little wider.

**Dr:** Wider scope.

**Pt:** Yeah.

**Dr:** So you get this anxiety from time to time and sometimes it gets worse but generally you'll have a certain level of anxiety. *[Recapping link between anxiety and somatic symptoms.]*

**Pt:** That's right.

**Dr:** So here we see several formats of the anxiety. One is clouding your vision or your thoughts, another is this dizziness, and another can be cramps or diarrhea.

**Pt:** Uh hmm.

**Dr:** So do you want us to explore this anxiety and what drives this anxiety? *[Recap, outlining treatment task.]*

**Pt:** Yes. Let's do that.

**Dr:** Because it sounds like it really torments you when it is there. *[Reflecting the torturous nature of his symptoms.]*

**Pt:** *[Sighs.]*

In this patient, unconscious anxiety was manifest as cognitive-perceptual disruption requiring anxiety reduction. In bringing down the anxiety you and he could both see that his somatic disturbances were a product of high anxiety. Through this work you are also able to build rapport, comfort the patient, instil confidence in your skills, gather history and diagnose the emotional linkage to the symptoms. All this took place in a 5-10-minute period at the beginning of this interview in this case.

In standard symptom based medical interviewing, just the process of thorough history taking can reduce some somatic symptoms through a similar process described above. Observe your patient's baseline state of unconscious anxiety and take note of shifts while you review his history. Summarize the findings and see if that helps further change his symptoms. This is likely one mechanism by which a traditional health professional assessment can be therapeutic.

### Recapitulation and Review

The technique of recapping is central to both anxiety reduction and verification of emotional drivers of PPD. Recapping is very much the same process as reviewing diagnostic and physical investigation findings with the patient. This review should include all data observed in terms of the linkages between feelings, anxiety, physical manifestations and mechanisms by which a person avoids feelings. This comprehensive review should be repeated to be sure the patient understands. Recapping is not only necessary to increase understanding and reduce symptoms, it is also a way for you to be able to better understand what has been observed. Recapping makes the next steps in the collaborative care process clear.

Patients with more smooth muscle and cognitive-perceptual disruption symptoms require more repeated and extensive recapping to replace these symptoms with self-reflection on affect and striated muscle anxiety. Here is an example of recapitulation with a patient who experienced cognitive-perceptual disruption during the psychodiagnostic evaluation. Recapping was done to reduce anxiety and build self-reflective capacity. When talking about a conflict he had with his boss, this man began to struggle to maintain his thought processes. He was staring blankly at me with signs of mental confusion and his voice was constricted. I now move to reduce anxiety.

**Dr:** Can you describe what happened in your body there for a second? *[Intellectual review to bring down anxiety.]*

**Pt:** I just...I just felt all lost.

**Dr:** Maybe ten seconds ago, what happened? Can you tell me what happened? *[Exploration of phenomena.]*

**Pt:** I just totally felt... everything blacked out... I almost.

**Dr:** Tell me what you noticed there. What did you experience in your head? *[Exploration of phenomena.]*

**Pt:** It was like a darkness that went up through my mind and I went all blank.

**Dr:** Okay, did your thoughts become jumbled? *[Exploring phenomena.]*

**Pt:** Very much. It just became all scrambled.

**Dr:** Okay, so how long did it last? Like a second or two? *[Exploring phenomena.]*

**Pt:** Seconds.

**Dr:** Okay, for a second you got that experience and then your thoughts were hard to sort out. Your thoughts blanked out. *[Recap.]*

**Pt:** That's correct.

**Dr:** Okay, so when we focused on underlying feelings, your anxiety went up and interrupted your thoughts. *[Recap.]*

**Pt:** That's right. It did.

**Dr:** Okay, so then was this interruption of your vision and thoughts triggered by the feelings you had? *[Recap linking feelings and symptoms.]*

**Pt:** Yes, it must be. Because you were asking how I felt toward my boss then all that happened right away. *[Hands starting to clench, takes a sigh: anxiety moving to striated muscle.]*

**Dr:** How is the anxiety now?

**Pt:** It has come down now.

**Dr:** Okay so this process can happen fast.

**Pt:** Yes.

**Dr:** Can we both watch it closely? Then we can bring down the anxiety by reviewing it when we need to? *[Setting the task of co-monitoring anxiety levels.]*

**Pt:** That sounds good.

**Dr:** So we see then that strong feelings can induce anxiety that can cause some specific symptoms including blurry vision and mental confusion. But these symptoms can be reduced just by examining them. *[Linking feelings anxiety and symptoms.]*

**Pt:** Yes, its like I'm afraid of those feelings. *[Hands firmly clenched and draws another sigh. Thought processes are clear.]*

**Dr:** So it's as if your mind manages those scary feelings by disconnecting your thought process and interrupting your vision. *[Further linking feelings anxiety and symptoms.]*

This is a patient who could not tolerate a high rise in anxiety. We see the physical impact of intellectual review in recapping: by intellectually reflecting the anxiety shifts into striated muscle and away from cognitive-perceptual disruption. As we focused on his symptoms and intellectually recapped, his anxiety is brought down to a manageable level. We can then verify with him that anxiety was interrupting his cognitive and perceptual field while building rapport and trust. Through this mobilization and recapping process, we confirmed together that anxiety was causing his specific functional neurological symptoms.

**Table 6.3: Interpretation of Results**

| Result | Interpretation and Action |
| --- | --- |
| Reduction in symptoms | If the symptoms are reduced or removed with an emotional focus, it strongly suggests that the symptoms were a manifestation of unconscious anxiety. |
| Rise and fall in symptoms in accordance with anxiety | If there is a rise and fall in symptoms in accordance with anxiety, it strongly suggests that there is a link between unconscious anxiety and symptoms. |
| No change in symptoms despite changes in anxiety | If there is absolutely no shift in somatic symptoms then it suggests that there are organic factors that are dominating the picture. Medical investigation or further interviewing is warranted. |
| Response that cannot be determined | An indeterminate response means that you cannot tell what the findings are and this suggests that there should be further focused interviewing. |

## Interpretation of Results

There are four possible outcomes from this psycho-diagnostic assessment (Abbass, 2005; Abbass, et. al., 2007).

1) Symptoms may be reduced or eliminated, suggesting strongly that the symptoms were caused by unconscious anxiety.

2) Symptoms may rise and fall during the interview in correlation with the degree of anxiety experienced, which also suggests a strong emotional factor.

3) There may be no change in symptoms suggesting that unconscious anxiety is not linked to the symptoms.

4) Indeterminate response where it is not possible to tell whether there is any linkage between unconscious anxiety and symptoms. This finding suggests that the procedure may need to be repeated or a short series of interviews provided.

This is much the same as an abdominal examination: in some cases, you need to repeat the palpation and press more firmly or in different areas. These possible results, interpretations, and recommended actions are outlined in table 6.3.

### When to Refer a Patient to Mental Health Services

Data from the psychodiagnostic interview may imply the patient should be referred for formal mental health care. The following findings should lead to considering such a referral:

1. *Psychotic phenomena*: Patients with fixed delusional ideas should be referred as this is a marker of a psychotic disorder presenting somatically. An example of this is a person who is convinced that he is being poisoned causing him physical symptoms.

2. *Suicidality*: Patients with active suicidal ideation in addition to somatic symptoms should be referred to mental health services.

3. *Substance dependence*: A person with active substance addiction may worsen with a rise in anxiety and is thus vulnerable to increased substance abuse without first addressing the addiction.

4. *Mania*: If a patient is showing signs of mania such as pressured speech, grandiose ideation, sleep disturbance, and impulsivity, a manic disorder is possible and a referral to mental health services is warranted.

5. *Prominent Dissociation*: Patients with prominent dissociation, with long memory gaps or fainting attacks should be referred to mental health services for management.

## CHAPTER 6 SUMMARY

■ *Patterns of unconscious anxiety include striated muscle anxiety, smooth muscle anxiety, and cognitive-perceptual disruption. Motor conversion is seen with a lack of striated muscle tension and paralysis.*

■ *Anxiety can be reduced by focusing on the body sensations, recapping on what has been learned and changing the area of focus.*

■ *By focusing on avoided feelings and observing physical and behavioral responses, it is possible to confirm a diagnosis of PPD in some cases and rule out such a cause in others.*

CHAPTER 7

# Modified ISTDP for the Health Professional

IF MEDICAL EVALUATION, PSYCHODIAGNOSTIC assessment, educational, cognitive and behavioral interventions do not result in adequate symptom relief, more in depth emotion-focused treatment sessions are warranted. We will herein review the basic ingredients and processes of ISTDP informed treatment sessions that can be applied in a primary care setting.

## Overview of ISTDP Informed Treatment Sessions

In this chapter, we review how to provide ISTDP theory informed treatment sessions. We review how to orient the patient, initiate the process, activate emotions and summarize the process afterward. We will also review some of the core emotional processes activated during the treatment. See table 7.1 for an outline. The method described here is an abbreviated version of the full ISTDP model that can be successfully applied in short treatment courses (Davanloo, 2005; Abbass, 2015).

## Knowledge Requirements for Providing These Sessions

ISTDP informed treatment sessions may be provided by a trained health professional who understands the theory and diagnostic technique described in the previous chapters. This process builds on the therapeutic relationship you have already established through evaluating and educating the patient. In order to provide these sessions, you must understand the core concepts described in chapters 5 and 6 as summarized in table 7.1.

### The Treatment Objective in a Nutshell

When combining these elements together, the objective is to help the person see 1) *how feelings that are mobilized in present life experiences are complex, 2) how these feelings are tied to past events, and 3) how they are manifest as increased somatic symptoms.* This statement contains the essence of how you will help your patients understand themselves. Of the unconscious feelings and impulses, the prime driver of somatic symptoms is guilt about rage. If these key concepts, tailored to the specifics of your patient, are repeatedly reviewed, even if only in brief

### Table 7.1:  Core Knowledge Requirements to Provide Modified ISTDP Sessions

**1.** The complex nature of unconscious feelings including loving feelings, grief due to losses, rage, and guilt about the rage.  All of these unprocessed feelings are seen in nearly all people with PPD.

**2.** The links between unconscious complex feelings, unconscious anxiety and defense mechanisms, including conversion and repression of emotions.

**3.** The link between past and present relationships, whereby feelings from previous relationships are mobilized in current relationships.

**4.** How to recognize the somatic pathways of unconscious anxiety and the process of motor conversion.

**5.** How to recognize the experience of feelings (grief, rage, guilt) versus somatic anxiety.

**6.** How to reduce anxiety by focusing on body cues and by reflecting on the interview process.

**7.** How to assess and handle the defenses against emotional experiencing by clarifying avoidant behaviors in the office and challenging these behaviors in concert with the patient.

**8.** How to recap and summarize the findings.

sessions over three or four meetings, many if not most, of your primary care patients will have significant symptomatic relief.

ISTDP has been studied and shown to be effective in treating a broad range of somatic symptom presentations including headache, back pain, fibromyalgia, pelvic pain/urethral syndrome, functional movement disorders, chronic pain, pseudoseizures, and mixed somatic presentations to the emergency department (Abbass, et. al., 2008; Abbass, et. al., 2009; Town and Driessen 2013; Russell, et. al., 2016). It was found to outperform mindfulness based stress reduction and controls in studies of patients with chronic pain (Chavooshi, et. al., 2016a and b). Treatment courses in these studies averaged from 3 to 16 treatment sessions. ISTDP has been found to be cost effective in about 15 studies through reductions in hospital costs, doctor costs, medications, and disability costs (Abbass and Katzman, 2013; Abbass, et. al., 2015; Russell, et. al., 2016). In addition, ISTDP has been effectively integrated into both emergency department and family medicine care of medically unexplained syndromes (Abbass, et. al., 2010; Cooper, et. al., in press).

## Step-by-Step Process for Sessions

These sessions should be structured much in the way a medical visit is structured.

1. *Orient:* Begin with an orientation of the process and a reminder to the person of what you and the patient understand about their problems already.

2. *Initiate the Process:* Ask the patient if he wants to examine how emotions impact his symptoms and to explore this together with you. Explore specific examples of times when symptoms, anxiety, or defense mechanisms occurred in detail.

3. *Mobilize Avoided Feelings:* Focus on the feelings and somatic sensations he had in those incidents.

4. *Observe the emotions* that are mobilized and how they impact the patient physically during the interview.

5. *Watch for signs* that he is bringing memories related to times in the past when he developed his patterns of handling complex feelings.

6. *Explore any past linked emotions* triggered by the process.

7. *Recapitulate on the findings* by linking together all the feelings, anxiety, defenses from the past to present relationships. Gather the patient's view on the process and findings.

8. *Plan further meetings* or follow-up.

In short, the process of these brief sessions is an expansion of what was described in the psychodiagnostic interview. The goal is further in depth understanding and awareness of how feelings impact the body. Another major goal is for the patient to develop empathy and compassion for himself as a person, for having experienced emotional wounds in his past and present life, and for having symptoms related to those emotional wounds. A third goal is to help the patient learn to experience feelings as opposed to developing somatic symptoms when feelings are activated. These sessions should always be concluded by thorough recapitulation and review of what has been learned to bolster the patient's capacity to battle against emotional avoidant patterns between meetings.

We outline these steps and provide case vignettes below.

## Orienting the Patient

In the previous chapters we reviewed how to evaluate your patient and how to perform a collaborative psychodiagnostic evaluation of emotional processes. Through this process you will have established rapport and trust with the patient and have determined that there appear to be emotions triggering physical symptoms. Thus, you and the patient are in agreement that there is a process of emotions making physical health worse. You both want to collaborate together to solve this problem. From this shared understanding, you can obtain consent from the patient to have some limited treatment sessions focusing on what these emotions are and how they impact current life experiences.

Orienting the patient to this specific treatment process involves 1) re-explaining your findings to the patient, 2) securing clear consent for a focused process of examining motions,

3) reviewing information collaboratively, and 4) establishing an open line of communication about every phenomenon that takes place while focusing on this emotional process in your office.

## Initiating the Process

After this orientation, the patient will be in one of four states of mind. When you identify these states of mind, you will know how to proceed. These states of mind are as follows:

### Anxiety

If the patient is experiencing obvious unconscious anxiety with hand clenching and sighing respirations, then a good place to focus is on what feelings are being mobilized while talking with you. This helps the person observe how his emotions are affecting his muscles and producing sighing respirations. It could also cue him to examine the moment and examine the emotional effect of being present in the office with you.

If anxiety is affecting the smooth muscle or the cognitive-perceptual field then the first approach is to bring down the anxiety by an intellectual review of the physical symptoms (table 6.1). This would bring more self-reflection on affect and shift anxiety to striated muscle resulting in a calming effect. Once the patient is calmer with striated muscle anxiety, you can proceed to focus on what emotions were being mobilized. This finding of anxiety in the smooth muscle and in cognitive-perceptual disruption suggests that a *graded format* of mobilizing feelings followed by intellectual review of the process should be undertaken to prevent an untoward increase in symptoms (chapter 8).

### Defenses

If the patient appears to be in a defensive position in terms of the manner of relating to you, then it is necessary to examine the defenses and help him recognize that even though he is consciously willing to examine emotions, some part of him is producing defenses and interrupting that process.

For example, if a person is extremely detached emotionally and sitting in the office avoiding you then it is important to point out that he appears to be detaching and help him see that this is going to get in the way of the goal of understanding how emotions work. If the person is in somewhat of a defiant position, then it would be important to further clarify if he wishes to examine emotional processes in the room. Questioning in the form of "Would you like us to look into what is happening?" will help to achieve this. The passive-compliant patient may sit there without any signs of anxiety but take such a passive role that the process will go nowhere. It is thus important to clarify the pattern of passively going along with you and clarify how this behavior stops the process of emotion activation: this clarification will undo this type of defense.

The medical parallel to this process is the patient with chest pain who comes for an examination. When you ask to examine his chest, he does not remove his shirt and will not allow you to take his blood pressure. To help the patient, you must be able to actually examine the chest. The same goes for emotional operations: defenses arise due to anxiety about the feelings. You have to clarify the blockages that don't allow you and the patient to understand his emotional processes. See "Interruption of Defensive Behavior" in chapter 6 for an example.

### Feelings

If the patient has activated complex feelings in the present and wishes to speak about these emotions then follow the patient to these emotions. For example, the patient may say "Yesterday I had an argument with my boss and I immediately got nauseated." You can focus on what feelings she has when she is talking about this incident. The patient may say she has anger and you can help her recognize and identify the physical component of anger. You can then follow this through to help her experience the anger and identify what other feelings are associated with this anger.

### No Signals

The fourth possible way a person can initiate the session is without any signals of anxiety, defense or feelings. The patient with no signals is usually not activated and engaged in the treatment process. In this situation, it is important to identify areas where they would like to focus and what the internal problems are that they are there to solve. In other words, take time to clarify the task and goals of the meeting. If it becomes apparent the patient is presenting in a passive way deferring to you to solve the problems, clarify the need for a shared process with the active involvement of the patient. These efforts will usually overcome passive compliance and allow feelings and anxiety to rise so you can proceed with a treatment session.

## Figure 7.1: **Treatment Session Algorithm**

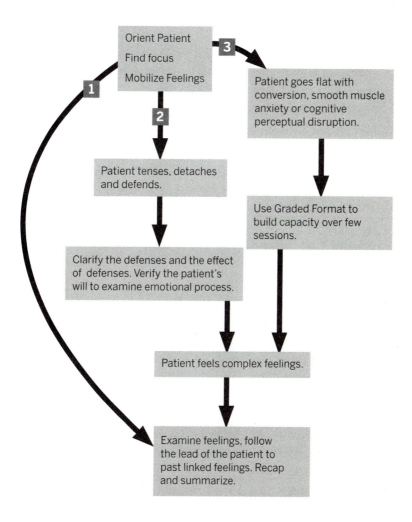

### Emotional Mobilization

With this collaborative therapeutic focus, the patient will inevitably respond in one of three different ways. The person will 1) feel feelings, 2) mobilize defenses and detach, or 3) goes "flat" with smooth muscle anxiety, conversion or cognitive –perceptual disruption. There is a treatment approach that you can use for each of these responses (see figure 7.1).

### Response 1. Feelings are Experienced

If a person is experiencing feelings such as grief about someone's death or anger and guilt about the anger towards someone in a recent incident, then you can follow these emotions and facilitate these experiences. You can conclude this segment by a review of the process to help the patient link these emotions to the physical symptoms they have been struggling with.

### Response 2. Defenses Rise

If the person becomes more emotionally detached from you, you can help him recognize that he is becoming detached, distancing and interrupting his own goal of understanding his own emotions and how these tie into his health problems. Thus, you can start to clarify and help him to challenge these emotionally detaching defenses. Thereafter, the emotions will eventually be experienced and you can help him go through the emotions and see any linkages to past complex feelings that are being stirred up in the office while talking with you.

### Response 3. Going Flat

If the person goes flat with smooth muscle anxiety, cognitive disruption, muscular weakness or a depressive response, then it is important to stop the process and intellectually recap on what has transpired. The goal at this point is to replace this repression of emotions with intellectualization and self-reflection about the emotions. Such self-reflective work will bring the anxiety into the striated muscle and this will bring a calming effect. The person will have a sigh or two and will feel more relaxed and solid (see chapter 6 smooth muscle). When they are calmer and able to self-reflect and anxiety is in the striated muscles, then you can increase the focus on underlying feelings once again. These are the characteristics of the graded format of ISTDP (see chapter 8).

### Feeling the Feelings

When the patient starts to feel an emotion such as grief, you can help her to experience the feeling. For example, you can say "You have a very painful feeling in you right now." This validation of emotions will help tears of grief to flow.

When unconscious violent rage is being experienced, the person will experience heat, energy and an urge to lash out in some way. At this point ask the person to paint a mental picture of the angry impulse that they are tending to hold back. This will allow you to see what the imagery is in their mind, and allow you and the patient to validate the rage. This imagery will also open the gates to other feelings and help you both understand why the rage is being shut down.

Once rage has been felt and expressed, guilt will be experienced about having such a buried urge, especially if that rage is toward a loved one. This guilt can be very strong as it is connected to the simultaneous experience of love and rage combined. This guilt is the main driver of PPD and self-destructive behaviors of all varieties: the patient lives like a criminal who must be restrained, shut down and punished. The essence of this therapeutic approach is to help the patient recognize that they have loved, they were emotionally wounded, and the normal emotional reactions of rage have been directed inward in the form of physical and/or mental health symptoms. This process will enhance self-directed compassion in a person who has been hurt and facilitate both symptom recovery and interpersonal relationship improvements.

### Explore Past Linked Emotions

When the emotions described above are somatically experienced, the anxiety and defenses will drop. The person will then be able to tie together current and past emotions. For example, they will link sadness, rage and guilt about the rage they have towards their husband to the same mixed feelings they had toward their father in the past. It is common for the type of emotional trauma to be similar, such as a husband and father who abandon them or who are controlling.

You can then guide the patient to help her to experience some complex feelings from the past. Throughout all this it is critical that you and the patient together are able to observe the process while exploring it. Thus, the process is a calm, collaborative exploration of these emotions in a safe and comfortable format.

## Recapitulate

After any experience of strong emotions, stop to recapitulate and review what has been learned. This should be done in a repeated fashion tying together the grief, the violent impulses attached to rage, the guilt about rage, the anxiety, the somatic symptoms, and the defense mechanisms used to cover the anxiety and emotions.

Say something like, "So did you notice when you felt this anger that your arm became strong and powerful with an urge to punch repeatedly? And as soon as you felt this urge to punch, an image of your father came to mind from a time when he had hurt you in the past. At that time in the past you had strong anger in your arm to punch and punch him repeatedly until he was badly damaged. And there is also a lot of guilt about that anger. It is as if you felt like you had actually done what you wanted to do in harming him. But did you notice however, the way this anxiety about these emotions was affecting you? Your arm was getting extremely tense at some points and also weak at other points. Do you think that this has to do with the urge that you had in your arm to punch your father? Do you think that you suppressed this rage because of your love for him?"

The patient may respond with her own recapitulation and fill in her own understanding of what has happened. This collaborative review is extremely important to improve her capacity to self-reflect about emotions in a manner that is compassionate toward herself. This process will lead to less repression of feelings and greater self-reflective capacity.

## Use the Therapeutic Relationship

If at any point when exploring emotional incidents outside of the office, the patient becomes very anxious, or goes flat with somatic symptoms, you can use the therapeutic relationship to examine what feelings are being stirred up. This examination will usually reduce symptoms and increase energy in the patient.

For example, if the patient develops a stomach upset when talking about his father in the past you can first bring down the anxiety by reflecting on the physical symptoms and then focus on what feelings were being stirred up towards you when talking about his father. This may at first seem like a strange thing to talk about for the patient. But the reality is that he walked in your office, you asked him about feelings and then he got stomach upset. Inevitably you are stirring strong feelings from the past because of your questioning, your attention and your concern for the patient: you are triggering attachment related feelings.

Focusing on these feelings toward you will reduce his fear of his own feelings and can bring a therapeutic experience of the avoided feelings. These feelings then will be linked to the attachments from the past. For example, the patient may perceive you as 'pushing hard' but after feeling the feelings with you, recalls clearly an incident when his mother pushed him against a wall to control him in childhood.

## The Complex Nature of Complex Feelings

Keep in mind that you are working with people who, out of guilt and fearfulness of harming others, develop symptoms, self-destructive mechanisms, anxiety and defenses as if they need to protect everybody from rage that they feel so guilty about. Hence, remember that all these mechanisms serve some element of a positive purpose. The unconscious mind is preventing the patient from doing harm to someone else by creating the symptoms. On the other hand however, all these mechanisms and symptoms have a destructive effect on the person. In sum, the patient is hurting himself and undermining your collective treatment efforts while protecting you from his aggression.

## Track Your Own Emotions

This engaged process will mobilize complex feelings in everyone, including you. It is important to recognize that you have feelings while you need to maintain therapeutic boundaries and intervene with empathy to explore your patient's complex feelings. It is often necessary to process your own feelings triggered during a session. Here are some suggestions for accomplishing this.

### Use Your Feelings as a Guide

You can use your reactions therapeutically to recognize that you are experiencing some parallel emotions along with the patient. This will allow you to empathize with the patient and know what they are feeling to some extent.

### Verify That Feelings are Being Felt

You can use your emotional reactions as a gauge to verify that your patient is actually experiencing his feelings versus just intellectually talking about them.

### A Breakthrough for Yourself

There may be a therapeutic benefit for you to contact feelings that may have been blocked at some points in life. If some feelings had not been previously experienced or worked through in your own current life or in the past, this may provide you with an opportunity to visit those emotions with compassion for yourself. Alternatively, you may find emotions are blocked in yourself suggesting you may consult a colleague for peer support or consult a therapist to work with your own unprocessed feelings.

### Prevent Burnout

Such work and focus in this type of approach can be protective against health professional burnout. As you can imagine, patients with multiple somatic symptoms will often stir up feelings of frustration and helplessness and related feelings in the health professional. Since none of us went into the health professions to be useless and be unable to help our patients, these feelings are important to recognize and process.

Many of us, if not most of us, went into health professions out of a conscious or unconscious wish to heal and help family members in our own past. Because of this drive to help and fear of being unhelpful, health professionals will react strongly to being in positions where they cannot help their patients. This feeling of helplessness is typical in clinicians trying to medically solve the somatic problems of patients with PPD. When PPD patients consciously or unconsciously resist treatment, further strong feelings are triggered toward patients and tied to past times of helplessness. This piling up of emotions, coupled with failure to optimally care of ourselves, is probably one of the central components of burnout in health professionals. Being aware of emotions and dealing with the emotional challenges of working with your patients can have a protective effect against these negative impacts of health professional practice (Crosskerry, et. al., 2010).

## The Central Role of Guilt

As noted above, guilt about rage is a central agent producing PPD and other self-destructive processes. Hence, help your patients recognize and feel guilt about any rage toward loved ones or others in the past. When they are able to do that, the anger turned inward is defused and the symptoms resolve. As they do this work, it is critical to help them access loving and forgiving feelings towards themselves, both related to the past and current times. In addition, they are usually able to feel loving feelings towards people for whom they have had buried rage in the past. This process is akin to forgiveness for oneself and also forgiveness of the other person to whatever degree is appropriate.

Hence, a shortcut approach to symptom reduction is as follows. When the patient is talking about anger and develops symptoms, you can ask them directly how they would feel if their anger had hurt that person. Such a question may seem a bit strange at first because the patient may not even have talked about harming the person, but on an unconscious level there is a violent rage and guilt about that rage present. Hence, she will quite typically feel some remorse right away when you point this out. This may rapidly and dramatically reduce symptoms within seconds or a few minutes within these interviews. These moments provide a great deal of diagnostic data as both you and the patient can see in real time the interplay between emotions and symptoms (Abbass, 2015).

## Initial Treatment Session:
## Moderately Resistant Patient

*The patient is a middle-aged man with chronic back and shoulder pain diagnosed with fibromyalgia on long-term disability. He arrived with anxiety evident with hand clenching and sighing respirations. The doctor focused on the anxiety he arrives with since this is a signal that strong feelings are activated. The anxiety in his muscles means he can tolerate focus on his feelings without worry about smooth muscle anxiety, conversion or cognitive-perceptual disruption interrupting the focus.*

> **Dr:** So I noticed that when you're coming in you're anxious. Is that something you observe yourself in your body? Do you feel anxious? *[Focusing on anxiety. Encouraging self reflection.]*
>
> **Pt:** Yeah. Just coming in here to meet with you today is, you know, a little stressful. *[Hands clenched]*
>
> **Dr:** What makes the tension in your body? What kind of feelings do you have that get stirred up just walking in to see me that gets your body tensed up like that? *[Focusing on underlying feelings.]*
>
> **Pt:** Why does it happen to me?
>
> **Dr:** Yeah, why do you get anxious? *[Focusing on underlying feelings.]*
>
> **Pt:** That's a good question. *[Laughs.]*
>
> **Dr:** Is that part of why you're here? *[Verifying his wish to explore emotional factors.]*

**Pt:** Yes, that's part of it. I get anxious and it's been going on for a couple of years, really.

**Dr:** Mm hmm. So what feelings do you have inside that get you tensed up just coming in the door? *[Focusing on underlying feelings.]*

**Pt:** I'm anxious, I don't know what to expect.

**Dr:** What emotions in you produce this anxiety? How else do you feel here with me apart from tense and anxious? *[Focus on underlying feelings.]*

**Pt:** *[Sighs]* How else do I feel?

**Dr:** Yeah.

**Pt:** I have no other feelings.

**Dr:** But you have lots of tension in you though, right?

**Pt:** Yeah.

**Dr:** What's driving underneath that? Why is that happening to you? *[Focusing on underlying feelings.]*

**Pt:** A whole lot of things in life that bother me and I guess I'm anxious about finding out some of them. *[Hands still clenching, sighs.]*

**Dr:** Let's see how we can figure some of that out together. *[Focusing on shared task of understanding his feelings.]*

**Pt:** Okay.

**Dr:** Why does that happen to a person like you that you get all that tension in you? What kind of emotions do you have underneath it right now, here with me? *[Focusing on underlying feelings.]*

**Pt:** Maybe the problems that I'm having aren't problems that I should be concerned about as much as I am? *[Sighs.]*

**Dr:** What feelings are underneath that anxiety? What are you shutting down? Why are you shutting yourself down? *[Focusing on underlying feelings. Clarifying the shut down of feelings.]*

**Pt:** I don't have any feelings. *[Sighs, hands clenching.]*

**Dr:** But you got a lot of tension instead. Why are you doing that to yourself? You get tension instead of feelings but why? What are the emotions that are in you that you're tense about? *[Linking feelings to anxiety. Focusing on underlying feelings.]*

**Pt:** Hmm.

**Dr:** We can look into that if you want us to look into that, to find what's beneath that anxiety. *[Verifying consent, undoing any defiance.]*

**Pt:** Well, that's why I'm here. *[Big sigh].*

**Dr:** Do you notice that you sigh? *[Pointing out anxiety in the form of muscle tension.]*

**Pt:** I think that I should be able to deal with things but I'm not. *[Self-criticizing.]*

**Dr:** You're putting yourself down in your mind. *[Clarifying defense.]* But, what feelings are causing that too? *[Focusing on underlying feelings.]*

**Pt:** I'm afraid I'm lost. What do you mean by how do I feel?

**Dr:** See, you have tension in your body but what feelings are within you? You get tense, but it's a mystery why's it happening to you.

**Pt:** Uh hmm.

**Dr:** Maybe we can figure that out together. Do you want us to try to do this together? *[Clarifying his will to focus on feelings.]*

**Pt:** That's basically why I'm here.

### Is it Okay to Focus on Feelings?

The process of emotional focus with patients at the point where anxiety and defenses are dominating can initially be confusing to the patient. The patient is unable to see beyond their symptoms to what feelings drive the symptoms because the entire process is not conscious at that time. As long as the patient has anxiety in the voluntary muscles and is thinking clearly and is willing to examine with you, continue to focus on what drives his anxiety and defenses.

> **Dr:** Okay, so what's underneath that? *[Focusing on underlying feelings.]*
>
> **Pt:** I think I'm scared of what I'm going to find out.
>
> **Dr:** What emotions do you feel here now? *[Focusing on underlying feelings.]*
>
> **Pt:** I feel angry.
>
> **Dr:** With who?
>
> **Pt:** I guess with me because I can't be angry with you. *[Turning anger inwards.]* I got no reason to be angry with you. *[Rationalizing.]*

## Handling Anger Turning Inward

Based on guilt about anger toward past attachment figures, it is very common for patients with PPD to direct anger inward. Much of these psychophysiologic symptoms are caused by self-directed rage due to guilt. To handle this, sustain focus on what mixed feelings they have in that moment that are turning inward. In this case I focus on the feelings that are being triggered toward me.

> **Dr:** You said you can't feel angry with me because there's no reason to feel angry with me and you say you get angry at you. Is that the way you deal with the anger? You get mad at you? Is that one of the problems you're having too? *[Clarifying the defense of self-attack.]*
>
> **Pt:** *[Sighs, sits forward.]* Yes, I do get self-critical. I'm a person who has always handled things, and done things and been able to handle things.
>
> **Dr:** Yeah.
>
> **Pt:** And there's things in my life now that I can't handle.

**Dr:** Uh huh. So, you're kind of getting critical of yourself and you say there's some anger in you but what you do is turn it all on yourself. *[Clarifying defense of self-attack.]*

**Pt:** I'm the only person to blame.

**Dr:** We're not talking about blame. We're only talking about feelings. You know when you feel hungry; it's a feeling in your body, right?

**Pt:** Right.

**Dr:** Now how does your body feel when you have this anger here? Do you feel anger or do you just get all tightened up when you feel anger? *[Linking feelings to somatic symptoms.]*

**Pt:** *[Hands clenching]* I get tense and I get sore. *[He links feelings to somatic symptoms.]*

## Linking Feelings to Symptoms

The initial focus on his underlying feelings is paying off. The effort to understand him on an emotional level has resulted in a stronger therapeutic alliance, and this helped him to see the links between his feelings and somatic symptoms. This prevented any debate or argument with the patient about the impact of underlying feelings on his somatic symptoms.

**Dr:** You get all sore?

**Pt:** My back.

**Dr:** You get pain in your back? It gets tightened up?

**Pt:** Yeah.

**Dr:** What feelings are underneath this tension in your body? One you say is anger. How does the anger feel? *[Focus on the experience of rage.]*

**Pt:** I just... *[Raises both arms in expressive fashion and no signs of tension. Some rise in somatic anger.]* Do you know what high blood pressure's like?

**Dr:** Yeah.

**Pt:** That's what I feel like.

**Dr:** Can you describe that in your body? Where's it at?
*[Focus on the experience of rage.]*

**Pt:** Through here (points to chest area, hands moving freely in expressive fashion) and my head. Up through my chest. *[Tension has left his body; somatic anger is present.]*

## Somatic Pathway of Rage

When complex feelings are activated, unconscious anxiety manifests primarily as striated muscle anxiety in this patient. However, when the somatic pathway of rage is activated, it displaces the unconscious anxiety and the person can now move freely and speak freely without undue anxiety in the vocal cords or tension constricting the arms. At this moment, there is usually a notable drop in somatic pain associated with muscle tension.

**Dr:** What feeling is it though?

**Pt:** Frustration.

**Dr:** Frustration with who?

**Pt:** With you. *[Smiling with mixed feelings present.]*

**Dr:** Okay, so you come in and you have some feeling of frustration in your body. Let's see how you felt there because what happened was you got all tensed up.
*[Linking feelings to anxiety, encouraging the experience of the rage.]*

**Pt:** Yeah.

**Dr:** Let's see if you can let the feeling get felt. Feel the feeling and not let it get all tightened up. Does that make sense? Feel these things and don't let tension take over.
*[Recap to help him differentiate anxiety from anger and to help him feel the anger.]*

**Pt:** Yeah.

**Dr:** How does that anger feel with me? How did you feel that in your body? *[Focus to experience the rage.]*

**Pt:** Like pressure and energy in my body trying to get outside. *[Freely moving arms. Tension has dropped as he is in contact with the rage.]*

**Dr:** Where is it at? *[Focus to experience the rage.]*

**Pt:** All through here *[points to chest area]*.

**Dr:** How do your arms feel when you felt anger? *[Focus to experience the rage.]*

**Pt:** My arms feel fine, other than... *[Makes two fists]*.

**Dr:** They feel like gripping, do they?

## Expressing the Rage: Portraying

When the patient is in contact with the rage, ask him to describe what it wants to do that he is ordinarily supressing and turning on himself. This allows you both to better understand the reasons he shuts himself down and develops symptoms rather than feeling the feelings.

**Pt:** Yeah, I want to grab hold of something. *[Grabbing and shaking motion.]*

**Dr:** Yeah. How would that be if that came out here with me? How would that be if you didn't control yourself and didn't shut down yourself like you did?

**Pt:** The anger wants to grab somebody or hit somebody.

**Dr:** How would they grab? *[Focus on the impulse.]*

**Pt:** Shake, like this. *[Grabbing and shaking motion.]*

**Dr:** If you didn't control them, what would they do? *[Focus on the impulse.]*

**Pt:** They'd want to be aggressive. They'd want to hit somebody.

**Dr:** How does that feel after you did that? What do you see me look like if you had done that?

**Pt:** I don't let my anger get the better of me and I just don't do that. *[Looks sad.]*

**Dr:** So you contain it all and you get a lot of tension, right? How would you feel if you had just come out and grabbed and beat on me just now?

**Pt:** I would have regretted it. *[Voice is choked up with guilt.]* I don't want to hurt you.

**Dr:** Uh huh.

**Pt:** And I would have regretted it. I would have been aggressive to you but not for any particular reason. I would be very upset with myself. *[Sniffles away tears of guilt.]*

## Link to Recent Losses

He went on to describe that his father was dying and had to move in with the patient for care. In addition, his young niece had terminal cancer.

**Dr:** What emotions do you have about all these things in your life going on, your father getting sick and soon dying, and your niece. We see you have a lot of mixed feelings triggered here with me making you tense. You hold the feelings in and tighten up. What feelings do you have with your father and niece? *[Recap and focus on feelings.]*

**Pt:** I can't do anything for my father. I'm helpless and hopeless. I mean I love my father dearly. *[Wave of grief with crying.]*

**Dr:** Mm hmm.

**Pt:** The last number of years we've gotten along better than we've ever gotten along in our lives and I don't want to lose him. *[Wave of grief with crying.]*

A moment later the grief passes.

**Dr:** So one thing is that you have sadness about the idea of losing your father. This painful feeling about losing him because it's been going well for the past few years. You're closer than you've been in the past.

**Pt:** If you grew up with my old man, he was a lead engineer.

**Dr:** Mm hmm.

**Pt:**  And he was a perfectionist. So everything had to be done just perfectly. He was very much a perfectionist in everything that he did. Very rigid and strict.

**Dr:**  Mm hmm.

## Past Linkage

He brought a past incident of mixed feelings with his father where he supressed intense rage and guilt about the rage.

**Pt:**  And I grew up with that and I used to hate him for years because of it.

**Dr:**  Is there some time you just had enough of him and you just felt furious with him?

**Pt:**  Yes, I recall once we were working together on a problem in the house and I was trying to help. I was twelve years old. The next thing I know he was yelling at me for using the screwdriver wrong. *[Hands start to clench.]*

**Dr:**  How do you feel toward him then?

**Pt:**  I wanted to punch him, pound him. *[Fist punches into other hand.]*

**Dr:**  How would you have pounded him?

**Pt:**  Right in his face! He'd fall over.

**Dr:**  So you punch him and he falls over?

**Pt:**  That's terrible.

**Dr:**  It's a terrible feeling.

**Pt:**  Yeah. *[Sniffles with painful feeling.]* He was so tough but now he's so weak. *[Tears of guilt and grief.]*

## End of Session Wrap Up

The patient noted that his pain had entirely left during the middle of this process. We were able to see he had been tensing up to block painful mixed feelings of grief, rage and guilt about rage toward the father he loved. From there we reviewed the treatment process.

**Dr:** So we see that you have a lot of mixed feelings with your father: rage and guilt about rage and love for him all at once. So the way these feelings were showing up was in the form of all this tension and self-criticizing here with me? Do you think that is what was happening? *[Recapping.]*

**Pt:** Yes. I felt very bad about having that old rage. I'm glad I've got this time left now with him. I'm gonna miss him very badly. *[Sadness returns, cries.]*

**Dr:** So what do you think about having a few more meetings to deal with any other feelings you have around this?

**Pt:** Yes, I'd like to do that.

**Dr:** So the main thing is to feel whatever feelings come up so the feelings don't go into muscle tension and pain. OK?

**Pt:** I'll aim to do that. Thank you, Doctor.

This initial interview included assessment of anxiety somatic pathways in addition to emotional focusing as described. It also included a review of his medical history, medications, and any psychiatric history.

### Third Treatment Session:
### Moderately Resistant Patient

*To illustrate a typical treatment session after the initial interview we review the third session of a young woman with headaches, choking sensations and body pain. She arrives reporting a conflict with her husband that led to anxiety and headache. She has unconscious anxiety with hand clenching and sighing respirations.*

**Pt:** Since last night I'm feeling very anxious and sore. I had a headache.

**Dr:** Anxious?

**Pt:** The tension is right here (shoulders and neck). *[Deep sigh and hands are clenching.]*

**Dr:**  Since last night? *[Focus to be specific.]*

**Pt:**  Yeah, Matthew and I had a bit of a fight.

**Dr:**  That came first or the anxiety came first? *[Focus to be specific.]*

**Pt:**  Yeah. All night and all day I've been feeling very, um, just tense.

## Decision Point

She has arrived with striated muscle tension and intellectualization about her conflict. Her anxiety is in a safe channel in the striated muscle and she is able to intellectualize about her feelings so I can safely focus on underlying feelings. This focus helps her feel the feelings and remove the somatic symptoms secondary to this anxiety.

**Dr:**  How do you feel toward Matthew? *[Focus to identify feelings.]*

**Pt:**  I'm not angry now, I don't... *[Deep sigh.]*

**Dr:**  You have tension, pain and anxiety though. *[Linking feelings to symptoms.]*

**Pt:**  I have tension though. I have a lot of tension right now.

**Dr:**  But, what do you feel besides anxiety? *[Focus on feelings.]*

**Pt:**  I mean, I guess I didn't identify it as anger.

**Dr:**  But is that how you feel?

**Pt:**  Yeah, it's anger.

**Dr:**  Uh-huh. What is it that tells you that you have anger inside you? *[Focus to experience the anger.]*

**Pt:**  Just the feeling of wanting to fight.

**Dr:**  How do you experience it, physically? What is it that tells you it's anger you're experiencing? *[Focus to experience the anger.]*

**Pt:**  Just instead of the anxiety or being anxious it kind of stops when I talk about it and get angry. *[Describes the rage displacing the unconscious anxiety.]*

**Dr:** Yeah, what do you experience physically that tells you it's anger, right now? *[Focus to experience the anger.]*

**Pt:** Just a physical rush of adrenaline rushing from my stomach up to my chest. *[Somatic pathway of rage, moves hands upward quickly.]*

**Dr:** Do you experience that right now though? *[Focus to experience the anger.]* Because some part of you wants to push that away and make you anxious instead. *[Clarification of symptoms versus feelings.]*

**Pt:** It was a split second. *[Snaps fingers, tension is low.]*

**Dr:** Yeah, in that split second how did you experience the rush? *[Focus to experience the anger.]*

**Pt:** It just came over me and I just... it was just.... *[Hands moving in expressive fashion.]*

## Portraying the Rage

This patient's reactions give enough data to show that she is feeling the rage: her tension dropped, her energy has increased, and she has an aggressive urge. With this data, I ask her what the avoided rage wanted to do that caused her to become so tense.

**Dr:** If this whole rage had blasted out of you, what way would this rage go if it came out in terms of your thoughts? *[Focus to portray the rage.]*

**Pt:** I would have been hitting him. *[Hand is in a fist and punching into other hand.]*

**Dr:** In what way though would this sense of an animal come out? *[Focus to portray the rage.]*

**Pt:** I would be hitting him on the head with my fist. *[Quietly punches one hand into the other.]*

**Dr:** What else? *[Focus to portray the rage.]*

**Pt:** On his chest.

**Dr:** On his chest. How much force is in you when you do this? *[Focus to portray the rage.]*

**Pt:**   A lot!

**Dr:**   What would you like to do to his head? *[Focus to portray the rage.]*

**Pt:**   Cut him with my rings.

## Guilt

A few minutes later, she is becoming visibly guilty with tears in her eyes.

**Dr:**   I sense you have a painful feeling about this rage inside, too. *[Focus to feel guilt.]*

**Pt:**   My Matt. *[Sobbing.]*

**Dr:**   For a split second there was real rage in there.

**Pt:**   Yeah.

## Link to Past Feelings: Transference

The patient feels guilty looking at the image of her battered boyfriend. The breakthrough of the feelings has removed the unconscious anxiety. Now her memory systems activate bringing a past link to her current mixed feelings.

**Pt:**   I had a picture of my father just now. I don't know why. *[Image from her memory.]*

**Dr:**   Uh-huh, how do you mean?

**Pt:**   He just came to my mind and I don't know why. I haven't thought about him for days.

**Dr:**   What makes him come to your mind right now? When you look at Matt's body, you mean?

**Pt:**   No, not when I looked at his body. Matt's body left my head, and then I saw my father. Just like a picture.

## Exploring Past Linked Feelings

Following this event, she had a clear memory of a situation with her father when she was eight. The impulse to harm the father by smashing his head and the guilt about this rage were identical to what she felt with her husband. It was around this age she started to develop headaches. At the end of the session she had no residual symptoms, and the body tension was gone. We recapped at the end of the session and educated her about the links to her symptoms.

> **Dr:** And you mentioned a headache too?
>
> **Pt:** Actually, yeah, I had a headache last night.
>
> **Dr:** Because all that anger was focused on the head of your father and Matthew too. To what extent are those all mechanisms to deal with the rage and the guilt? *[Clarification of sympathy symptoms; her headache is linked to urge to damage loved ones' heads.]*
>
> **Pt:** I never thought of it that way. But, yeah, that makes a lot of sense, but right now I feel a lot of relief.
>
> **Dr:** There's no headache now.
>
> **Pt:** There's no headache. My back's not sore. My muscles are relaxed. I'm not tense here or here. *[Points to stomach and chest.]* My stomach muscles are loose.
>
> **Dr:** So the feelings seem to have manifest as a lot of pain symptoms since last night. As if you battered your father and husband and have to suffer over that. You pounded their heads and bodies then you get pain on your head and your body.

## Summary

Here we see the process of helping her feel the feelings she was anxious about. When she came in contact with the anger, the anxiety reduced and she was able to describe the impulse. When she felt the rage, she had guilt about the anger as if she had done violence. Right after this her mind linked the buried feelings with her father to those with her husband.

**Dr:**  So we saw the link between old feelings, anxiety and symptoms today.

**Pt:**  It's clearly related to my body symptoms, for sure.

**Dr:**  What do you think about meeting back a few more times to see what happens in between and see how you manage things?

**Pt:**  That sounds good.

## Planning of Future Meetings

At the end of these brief meetings, the patient and you will have a better understanding of emotional processes and their impact on health. The decision then can be made whether the intervention has been adequate in reducing symptoms and increasing understanding. You might agree to add further sessions or to intensify treatment if there is a limited response, no response, or some sign of worsening. Otherwise, it may be necessary to refer a patient to a therapist for more in depth treatment sessions.

## The Highly Resistant Patient

The more resistant and defensive patient tends to avoid both his feelings and the therapist. Typically, these defenses are entirely unconscious to the patient: he doesn't know he is guarding his abdomen when you try to examine him. The vignette in chapter 6 and others (see Abbass, 2015; Abbass, 2016) show examples of how to clarify and challenge defenses to allow some feelings to be experienced.

The process of handling defenses involves careful clarification of what you observe and the impact it is having on the goals of the session. Thus, it is an educational moment to help the patient see what he is doing so he can correct himself and do the best for himself and his health.

When you evaluate your patient, you must decide whether you and she can access her emotions or whether the defenses are so tightly held that your treating relationship could be compromised by trying to help her stop defending. Hence, be careful when you meet resistance since your first priority as a health professional is maintaining a trusting treatment relationship. If you cannot help your patient stop defending enough to diagnose PPD as illustrated in chapter 6 then a referral to another therapist may be needed to help her access her underlying feelings.

### Cautionary Notes

In conducting these emotionally activating treatment sessions, the clinician should be aware of specific issues or events that could result in some worsening of the patient's situation or put the patient/clinician relationship at risk.

### Depression and Suicidal Ideation

It is important to note that rage directed inward on an unconscious level can activate major depression. The main manifestations of this may be physical fatigue, drop in mood, vegetative signs of depression and suicidal ideation. As a general principle, patients with active suicidal ideation should not be treated by a primary care health professional, as they should be urgently referred to mental health services. If during treatment sessions there are signs of deepening depression, consideration should be given of referral and consultation with a mental health professional.

### Paranoid Ideation

If a patient appears to develop paranoia manifesting as extreme fear or delusional ideation, a mental health referral is also warranted. Sometimes, the first manifestation of a psychotic disorder is somatic symptoms or somatic delusions. One example of this is a patient convinced despite repeated reassurance, that there are insects under his skin. Often it will take more than one meeting for paranoid ideation to become clear.

### Development of New Physical Symptoms

If your patient develops new somatic symptoms in treatment sessions, this may reflect an organic process requiring medical care. For example, if you are working with a patient who you felt to have irritable bowel syndrome and the patient develops new symptoms including severe pain, rectal bleeding, or other signs that do not fit the standard picture of irritable bowel syndrome, make appropriate referrals and suspend the treatment sessions. It may be that the patient had an inflammatory process, or another medical condition, or that there is a combination of a PPD and a medical disorder.

## CHAPTER 7 SUMMARY

■ *When patients do not respond to educational, cognitive and behavioural interventions, an emotion focused process based on Intensive Short-term Dynamic Psychotherapy (ISTDP) maybe helpful.*

■ *Steps for an ISTDP informed treatment session include orientation, selecting a focus, emotional mobilization, identification of emotions, reviewing findings, and planning.*

■ *With active emotional focus, patients will feel their feelings, defend and distance from the interviewer or 'go flat' with the development of smooth muscle symptoms, conversion or cognitive-perceptual disruption.*

■ *These patterns dictate how the treatment process can proceed. Patients with severe depression, paranoia, or worsening symptoms should be referred to mental health services.*

CHAPTER **8**

# The Graded Format of ISTDP

PATIENTS WHOSE COMPLEX FEELINGS convert into smooth muscle anxiety, depression, conversion or cognitive-perceptual disruption require a process to build capacity to tolerate anxiety. As described briefly in the psychodiagnostic section (Chapter 6), this process involved cycles of focus to identify underlying feelings alternating with recapitulation (see figure 8.1).

When anxiety is in the striated muscles and the person is self-reflecting, pressure to identify feelings can safely be applied but when anxiety is on other channels recapitulation is needed to build the capacity to self-reflect. This reflective process converts anxiety to striated muscle and allows the person to feel and process the feelings safely. This graded process raises the threshold at which a patient develops somatic symptoms: hence, it improves overall function.

### Dealing With Repression: **Using Graded Format**
*The following vignettes are of a 30-year-old man with severe irritable bowel syndrome and major depression (adapted from Abbass and Bechard, 2007; and Abbass, 2015). In the consultation, he developed reflux symptoms and abdominal cramps at a low rise in feelings reflecting poor anxiety tolerance.*

**Figure 8.1: Graded Format**

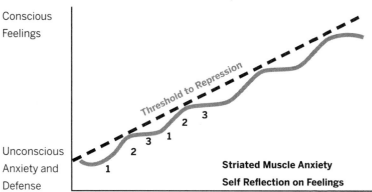

1. **Focus on feelings**
2. **Rise in complex feelings and anxiety**
3. **Recap to bring self-reflection and striated muscle anxiety**

**Dr:** Can you tell me about a time you experienced this stomach upset and diarrhea?

**Pt:** It comes out of the blue. There is no warning. *[Suggests he does not see emotional linkage.]*

**Dr:** Can you describe a specific time this happened so we can see how that works? *[Focusing to be specific.]*

**Pt:** It happened when I missed the first session.

**Dr:** Can you tell me about that? How did you feel when you missed the session? *[Focus to identify feelings.]*

**Pt:** I called you then got cramps and later diarrhea.

**Dr:** When you called me how did you feel? *[Focus to identify feelings.]*

**Pt:** I thought I was an idiot for missing the meeting.

**Dr:** You mean you were angry... but at who? *[Focus to identify feelings.]*

**Pt:** I am an idiot for missing it.

**Dr:** So, you mean angry at yourself? Is that what happens at times? *[Clarifying defense of turning anger inward.]*

**Pt:** Yes, I guess it does.

**Dr:** Because when you told me about that you became angry at yourself? *[Recap on defense of turning anger inward.]*

**Pt:** Yes, I did.

**Dr:** Can we look into that? How that happens here? *[Focus on task and patient's will.)*

The doctor hears gurgling sounds but the patient looks completely relaxed with no striated muscle tension. This is suggestive that his anxiety is not directing to the striated muscle and is rather being repressed into the smooth muscle of the GI tract: the patient looks "relaxed" but the GI tract is very active.

**Dr:** What is happening now?

**Pt:** Heartburn. *[Points to his chest.]*

**Dr:** Did you just get heartburn? Anything else?

**Pt:** I can hear my stomach gurgling.

**Dr:** So you can hear it gurgling. Is this what happens sometimes when you have strong feelings and anger, that you get heartburn and cramps? *[Recap linking feelings with anxiety and somatic symptoms.]*

**Pt:** Yes, it must be.

**Dr:** Because in your approach to talking about anger you got heartburn and cramps here. So is that where the anger goes? *[Repeat recap.]*

**Pt:** Must be, because it just happened!

This is evidence that repression of emotions took place into the smooth muscle. To confirm this finding and to ascertain the level of anxiety intolerance he had, the process is repeated with another focus.

**Dr:**  Can you tell me about another time that this happened? *[Focus to specific incident.]*

**Pt:**  Yes, when I'm angry with my brother, I don't say anything. I ignore him.

**Dr:**  Can you tell me about a time that happened? *[Focus to specific incident.]*

**Pt:**  Yes, just the other day he did something to irritate me... and that is coming back again.... the heartburn.

**Dr:**  So again, when you speak of anger, your stomach reacts with acid and cramps. *[Recap linking feelings with anxiety and somatic symptoms.]*

Again, the patient looks totally relaxed with no striated muscle response but the anxiety is affecting the smooth muscle in his GI tract. This suggests that at a low rise in anxiety he develops smooth muscle anxiety. He has severe repression manifest as severe irritable bowel syndrome with symptoms developing with low levels of anxiety. See figure 8.2.

**Figure 8.2: Threshold to Repression**

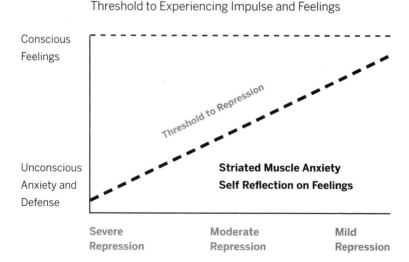

Threshold to Experiencing Impulse and Feelings

Conscious Feelings

Threshold to Repression

Unconscious Anxiety and Defense

**Striated Muscle Anxiety**
**Self Reflection on Feelings**

Severe Repression          Moderate Repression          Mild Repression

Thus, we confirmed that a direct effort to mobilize the unconscious feelings as seen in chapter 7 would likely result in a worsening of his GI symptoms as the threshold to repression was passed. We conclude this session and set a shared task to understand how his emotions affect his stomach over a series of sessions.

> **Dr:** So, what if we have some meetings to focus on how these feelings affect your stomach and your mood?
>
> **Pt:** Okay. That sounds like a good idea.
>
> **Dr:** Maybe you can try to notice when that happens during the week and we can focus on it here.

### Case Vignette: 4th Session

*This vignette is from the 4th session after he had some improvement in anxiety tolerance.*

> **Dr:** So when you were coming in today, you noticed some stomach upset?
>
> **Pt:** I was thinking about this anger thing and was upset with my brother the other day. *[Has a partial sigh indicating some striated anxiety.]*
>
> **Dr:** So there were some strong feelings you came to speak about and your stomach reacted. Do you have any cramps or heartburn now? *[Recap linking feelings with anxiety.]*
>
> **Pt:** No not now. *[Hands are somewhat clenched indicating striated muscle activity.]*
>
> **Dr:** Can we look into the feelings you have coming in today? *[Focus to identify underlying feelings.]*
>
> **Pt:** I was at his place and we were talking about growing up. He seemed to think it was a perfect childhood and I felt annoyed at him. *[Isolating affect, intellectual response with no body response.]*

**Dr:** How do you experience your anger? *[Focus to identify feeling.]*

**Pt:** I got nauseated and had diarrhea after.

**Dr:** So the anger again went to your stomach? *[Recap linking feelings with anxiety.]* Why didn't you get to feel the anger? What were you afraid of? *[Focus on anxiety.]*

**Pt:** I don't know *[burping]*. I'm getting cramps again now. *[Points to abdomen indicating smooth muscle anxiety.]*

At this point the anxiety is above the threshold of his tolerance. Continuing in this direction would lead to increased smooth muscle anxiety so instead we stop and recap.

**Dr:** So right now the anger we focus on goes to cramps. Is that process happening again? *[Recap linking anger and anxiety.]*

**Pt:** Yes.

**Dr:** So when we focus on the feelings now, the emotions go to your stomach rather than being felt. *[Repeat recapitulation.]*

**Pt:** Yes.

**Dr:** Can we look at what is happening here with me as we talk? How you are feeling here with me when we speak? *[Change of focus to the relationship in the room.]*

To reduce the anxiety, you can focus on body responses, recap or change focus (see table 6.1 for anxiety reducton techniques). If one approach does not work to reduce anxiety, then another one will work.

**Pt:** With you? I don't have any feelings with you. I feel mad at myself. My stomach still feels a bit bad. *[Not showing any striated anxiety meaning that anxiety is in the smooth muscle.]*

**Dr:** So again, when the emotions rise, anger turns inward on yourself. As if you are shutting down the anger, to hold it inward and keep it away from any one else. *[Recap feelings, anxiety and defense.]* How would you feel if you had been angry in some way with your brother or here with me?

Note this is primarily an intellectual question but alludes to the reason he uses repression and attacks himself: fear of rage and guilt about doing harm to others. It helps him intellectually see that he cares about others and doesn't want to do harm. This type of focus can improve his anxiety tolerance and reduce his fear of feeling rage, thus overcoming repression.

**Pt:** It would feel pretty bad. He has had a pretty tough time for the past 5 years since Mom died and his marriage was in trouble too. He has the same thing I do with the bowel and anxiety. *[Empathic response, albeit intellectual.]*

**Dr:** So there is positive feeling as well. Is this why the anger turns inward on yourself? To protect him? *[Recap linking complex feelings with defenses.]*

**Pt:** To beat up on me... I feel always like I should be punished for some reason...or that someone will punish me. *[Demonstrating understanding of the dynamic.]*

**Dr:** This is very important. So you have love at the base, but anger as well. When the anger comes, it is shut down into depression, anxiety, and some kind of guilt system? Like as if you had harmed someone you care about? *[Recap linking complex feelings with anxiety and defense.]*

**Pt:** ...so direct it at myself? *[Contributing to the recap.]*

**Dr:** Do you think?

**Pt:** Seems that way to me. It makes sense but I don't want that anymore. *[Looks stronger, calmer and has striated signals back with better body tone, hands clenched.]*

**Dr:** Let's see what we can do about it. *[Pressure to active focusing.]*

**Pt:** I'm not sure what to do. *[Some tension, sigh.]*

**Dr:** How do you feel toward me right now? *[Pressure to identify feelings.]*

**Pt:** Frustrated.

**Dr:** How do you feel this frustration inside? *[Focus to identify feelings.]*

**Pt:** I don't. It is toward me really.

**Dr:** So back at you again? Let's see how we can address that, to stop it. Because the feelings go in a few directions... to your stomach, to anxiety, to depression, to avoidance and to a passive position. All back on yourself... as if to protect the other person. *[Recapitulation and Focus to identify feelings.]*

**Pt:** That is what I'm doing, and I don't like it really....

By this point in the session, he shows more energy, less smooth muscle discharge, and has some access to striated muscle anxiety and self-reflection on affect. These are typical early treatment responses in ISTDP therapy when the process is going well with a person with severe repression. And this is often to your own pleasant surprise after seeing the patient look the same, with the same health complaints for years despite treatment efforts. Looking at figure 8.2, the patient is now in the section of moderate repression, still with the potential to have GI smooth muscle responses but at a higher threshold than before. That is, he can tolerate a higher level of complex feelings without going over threshold. This moves him closer to being able to experience his underlying feelings, the ultimate goal of the process. The patient can now begin to think and talk about his emotions without exacerbation of his symptoms.

## Case Vignette: 8ᵗʰ Session

**Pt:** I have been feeling better... the diarrhea has stopped for a few weeks now, but I've been noticing I don't like my sister-in-law very much. *[Striated anxiety with hands clenching and he has a sigh.]*

**Dr:** Can you tell me more about that? First why your diarrhea has stopped.

**Pt:** I'm not sure exactly *[sighs]* but something is different. I am thinking about the feelings more and not letting them get to me... the anger and anxiety thing we talk about.

Here we see signs of better capacity to self-reflect and anxiety is in striated muscle. These changes correlate with reduction in smooth muscle anxiety and repression: he now is on the mild repression side of figure 8.2 with higher anxiety tolerance.

**Dr:** Can we look into what happened with your sister-in-law? A specific situation you noticed.

**Pt:** Yes, my nephew John's gerbil died and she wanted to flush it down the toilet... my nephew was so upset and crying.

**Dr:** How did you feel? *[Focus to identify feelings.]*

**Pt:** I told her to be sensitive and consider the effects on John... and she did. *[Sighs again.]*

**Dr:** She had a good response to that?

**Pt:** Yes, she did actually. She was surprised I said anything and she thanked me for it later. What I said was measured and calm. I was a bit surprised! *[Proud and smiling at his new-found assertiveness.]*

**Dr:** So you felt good about that and good with her too? *[Clarification and Pressure to positive feelings.]*

**Pt:** Yes, but when she was saying that it tore my heart out and I felt enraged. *[Sighs and emergence of next component of the complex feelings.]*

**Dr:** How do you physically experience the rage when you think of it now? *[Focus to experience the rage.]*

**Pt:** It just... *[Moves hands from lower abdomen to upper body in sweeping motion, indicating somatic pathway of rage is beginning to activate.]*

**Dr:** How does that feel now? *[Focus to experience rage.]*

**Pt:** Its in my stomach and chest... moving up... a heat. *[Tension is now dropped and patient is energized with some degree of somatic pathway of rage activated.]*

**Dr:** How does that feel? *[Focus to experience rage.]*

**Pt:** Like I want to poke, to point. *[Gestures in a strong fashion.]*

Now that he is experiencing some of the rage, I ask what it wants to do in terms of his imagination.

**Dr:** How does it want to come out if it is not stoppable?

**Pt:** It wants to zap out like a laser beam. *[Forceful and expressive.]* And it would zap her into the wall.

**Dr:** Then what happens?

**Pt:** Then she is stopped.... And I feel bad. *[Tears form in his eyes.]*

**Dr:** It's a very painful feeling... *[Resonating with his guilt.]*

**Pt:** Yes. *[Weeps quietly with some guilt about the rage.]*

It is important to note that at this point, anxiety and defenses are temporarily absent. After the wave of guilt passed it is time again to recap. With the experience of feelings, it is typical that past linked feelings come to mind where the patient originally had interrupted attachments.

**Dr:** So in that moment, there were strong complex feelings all at once. You identified with John and his loss and this mobilized sadness and a degree of rage in your body. But this rage had guilt attached to it.

**Pt:** Yes. But I didn't get diarrhea or cramps that time, and I said something. It worked out well really.

**Dr:** Yes, you were conscious of the feelings at that time but didn't get to quite experience them until now. And when you did feel them, the anxiety and tension dropped and the feelings were felt. But the feelings were mixed and strong. Before, it would have been to the washroom and a panic, maybe becoming more depressed, but for sure not talking about it. *[Recap, linking feelings, anxiety and defense.]*

**Pt:** That is for sure.

**Dr:** But we have a question about these feelings. Do you have any thoughts what this all meant to you and why you felt so strongly?

**Pt:** I do *[wells up with wave of sadness and tears]...* My Mom *[Therapeutic alliance brings link to a past figure with whom there is unresolved emotion].*

**Dr:** There is a very painful feeling... *[resonating and highlighting].*

**Pt:** *[Weeping]* My father and mother divorced when I was 5 years old. All I remember after that was how I was not allowed to talk about my father and rarely got to see him. My mother wouldn't allow it. It was like he died.

**Dr:** There is a lot of painful feeling there.

**Pt:** *[Crying, as more grief arises].*

In the opening minutes of the session we see a common response in patients while being treated with ISTDP. The therapy is bringing changes at an unconscious but not at a conscious level. Patients will often report feeling better, having more awareness of emotions, but not being able to explain why things are better or exactly what has changed. However, knowing the different discharge pathways of unconscious anxiety, you can understand why his smooth muscle symptoms have stopped.

## CHAPTER 8 SUMMARY

■ *Patients who go 'flat' at a rise in complex feelings need assistance to build anxiety tolerance and self-reflective capacity.*

■ *A graded format comprised of cycles of recap and emotional focus can build anxiety tolerance.*

■ *When patients can self-reflect on emotions, the anxiety shifts from other pathways into striated muscle.*

■ *This capacity building step makes later emotional experiencing both possible and safe while overcoming symptoms including conversion, smooth muscle anxiety and cognitive- perceptual disruption.*

CHAPTER 9

# Synthesis and Conclusion

UNDERSTANDING HOW EMOTIONS and emotional attachments affect brain-body pathways is crucial to the practice of health care. Psychophysiologic disorders develop from important events that, by affecting neural mechanisms, determine how stress affects minds and bodies. We have described a step-by-step process for evaluating psychophysiologic disorders, explaining them to patients and providing educational, cognitive, behavioural, and emotional treatment components. Figure 9.1 outlines an approach to using these steps to treat these common conditions in a primary healthcare setting.

## Process for Evaluation, Education, and Treatment of PPDs

### Step 1: Medical Evaluation

As described in chapter 2, a through history and physical plus targeted laboratory tests and imaging studies are necessary in the evaluation of all patients. By clearly separating pathologic conditions from psychophysiologic conditions, not only can a structural disorder be ruled out—thus reducing the need for expensive and sometimes invasive medical treatment—but the clinician can rule in a PPD that can be effectively treated. Patients with unexplained medical symptoms are likely to have a psychophysiologic disorder, especially if they have had other PPD-like symptoms, a history of traumatic life events, a compatible personality profile, and present-day stressful situations that activate their symptoms. By confirming the diagnosis of a PPD, the clinician can initiate a series of interventions to help the patient resolve the symptoms. Since it is possible for most patients to completely recover, they can begin to shed feelings of frustration, stigma, and shame as soon

**Figure 9.1 Synthesis**

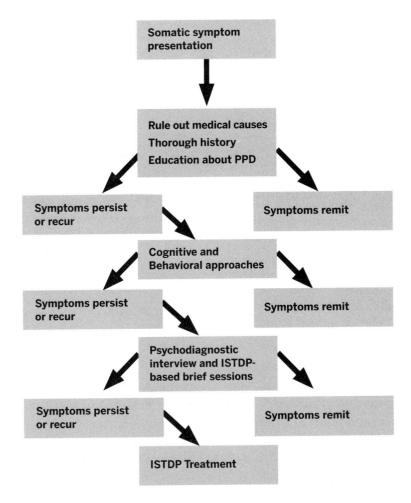

as the diagnosis is made. Through understanding how stress and symptoms can cause and perpetuate symptoms, many patients will develop hope and find the courage to face their symptoms, their emotions, and the situations in their lives that trigger or perpetuate symptoms. A minority of patients will achieve dramatic recoveries from PPD simply by being given this diagnosis.

The process of providing care usually leads to trust. If the patient is resistant to or does not understand the diagnosis of a PPD, there is the danger of losing rapport. Since trust is critical to helping patients with PPD, the provider should make this the first priority. More investigation of the patient's symptoms and more explanation may be necessary. It may be helpful for the patient to read about the mind-body connection (see appendix for resources) and return for follow up visits. The emotion-focused diagnostic interview described in chapter 5 demonstrates the connections between emotions and physical symptoms in real time. Making that connection helps patients understand the underlying nature of their symptoms.

### Step 2: Education, Cognitive, and Behavioral Interventions

In chapters 3 and 4, we described the roles of educational, cognitive, and behavioral approaches to improve the patient's ability to actively calm the mind and body and to become less reactive to symptoms. Clinicians can help patients understand that they are not diseased and that their symptoms are the result of learned neural pathways. We describe a number of cognitive and behavioral methods to help patients. These include reducing fear of the symptoms, taking control over them, being more active, challenging triggers to symptoms, practicing meditative exercises, recognizing the relationship between emotions and symptoms, expressing emotions in writing and in conversations, emphasizing compassion for self and others, and taking actions to alter stressful life situations. These approaches can be accessed by self-guided recovery programs using available printed and online resources (see appendix) and can be facilitated by medical and mental health care providers. Clinicians can point patients to these resources and reinforce these concepts while monitoring their progress in brief office visits. Some health care providers will develop skills in emotion-based therapy, while others will refer patients who need more care to trained counsellors.

### Step 3: Psychodiagnostic Evaluation and Brief ISTDP-based Sessions

Physiology of emotions and approaches to help a person identify and feel emotions were reviewed in chapters 5 - 8. With clinical experience those who use this approach can facilitate the resolution of symptoms in a range of patients who do not respond to the more conservative measures in steps 1 and 2. This further step requires an understanding of unconscious emotional processes and practice over time to develop skills. Many seek support while learning the process. We outlined cautions that the clinician needs to be aware of when undertaking this type of therapy.

### Step 4: ISTDP Treatment

For more complex or resistant patients not responding to the above steps, a formal course of a treatment such as ISTDP is warranted. This treatment can address the majority of patients with persistent or recurrent PPD-related symptoms. In chapter 7, we reviewed issues of patient selection and safety when using this model. Finally, in chapter 8 we reviewed a graded approach to build anxiety tolerance for patients with prominent repression or fragile character structure.

### When to Refer

Persistent symptoms may point to an underlying medical condition. Organic factors should be kept in the differential list until symptoms abate. Certain medical signs and symptoms should trigger further investigations and/or referrals to medical or surgical specialties.

Non-response to any of these steps maybe an indication for referral to mental health services or specialty psychophysiologic disorders services. You may have inadequate time, training, or comfort level to manage some patients. Over time you may build skills to work with more complex or resistant cases.

### Additional Resources

There are a variety of written materials and course offerings that can help you learn more about PPD and its treatment. Video recording based training courses and supervision in ISTDP are offered around the world. Periodic courses in other PPD treatment approaches are likewise offered widely.

## CHAPTER 9 SUMMARY

■ *A model for the treatment of PPD is presented.*

■ *It is essential to make an accurate diagnosis to both rule out a structural disorder and rule in PPD.*

■ *Education about PPD is the cornerstone of treatment.*

■ *A variety of cognitive and behavioral interventions can be offered to the patient.*

■ *A psychodiagnostic assessment can be performed to uncover direct connections between emotions and PPD symptoms.*

■ *ISTDP can be undertaken by the health professional to access emotions and reduce symptoms.*

■ *Referral to specialists in ISTDP may be necessary for some patients.*

# Appendix

### List of Evidence to Review in the Diagnosis of PPDs:

#### History

**Onset:**

*Did symptoms begin in association with a physical injury or not?*
Symptoms that arise upon awakening from sleep are often PPD.
Symptoms that occur without a specific injury are often PPD.

*If in relation to an injury, have symptoms persisted after the time in which healing would occur?*
Symptoms that persist after sufficient time for healing are often PPD.

*Did symptoms occur in association with particular stressful life events?*
Symptoms that begin in association with emotional conflicts are often PPD.

#### Description:

*Do symptoms fit the distribution of nerve lesions or other known anatomical patterns?*
PPD symptoms often do not conform to known distributions, but rather are seen in large areas, such as one side of the body, or the whole arm, leg, hand or foot. PPD symptoms are often symmetric, which is unusual for specific nerve lesions.

*Do symptoms come and go or vary in intensity greatly?*
Symptoms that "turn on" and "turn off" at random intervals are often due to PPD.

*Are there specific triggers for symptoms that do or do not fit with structural relationships?*
Triggers are experiences that trigger the brain to activate PPD symptoms. Movements, foods, light, sounds, temperature, and weather changes are common triggers. Often PPD symptoms are triggered inconsistently which is a clue to the diagnosis. Even when triggers consistently lead to symptoms, if the triggers do not fit with a structural diagnosis, this may be a clue to PPD. For example, sitting leading to back pain that occurs in certain chairs consistently, but not in other chairs.

*Do the symptoms shift from one body region to others?*
*Have the symptoms spread to adjacent areas over time?*
Symptoms due to PPD often move from one area to another. Pain or paresthesias may occur for some time in one body region, then disappear as the symptom shifts to another area. Symptoms that begin in one area then spread over time to adjacent areas are often due to PDD.

*Are symptoms subjective?*
Pain, paresthesias, fatigue are symptoms that can be created by the brain.

**Past History and ROS:**
*Does the patient have a history of other syndromes that are commonly seen in association with PPD?*
People with PPD often have a history of a wide range of disorders that are often due to PPD, such as IBS, fibromyalgia, anxiety, depression, fatigue, headaches, etc.

*Does the patient have a history of early life adversity?*
Early life adversity often primes or sensitizes the danger/alarm mechanisms of the brain, thus laying the groundwork for PPD in the future.

**Personality Traits:**
*Does the patient have a history of perfectionism, goodism, self-sacrificing, overly conscientious, guilt, low self-esteem, responsible for others, not standing up for self?*

Individuals with these characteristics are likely to put extra pressure on themselves. This can lead to an increased likelihood of developing PPD.

### Physical Examination:

*Are symptoms reproducible with specific movements that fit with a structural explanation?*
Pain that is associated with significant limitation, such as of the hip joint, is often not due to PPD, while pain that occurs without loss of range of motion is more likely due to PPD.

*Is the physical exam normal with respect to objective findings, e.g., neurological exam?*
Normal neurological exams make PPD more likely, while an abnormal neurological exam points to a structural process.

### Testing:

*Do lab and imaging tests reveal clear evidence of structural disorder?*
Evidence of a tumor, fracture or infection rules out PPD. On the other hand, negative testing in the face of significant symptoms suggests PPD.

*Are the positive findings commonly seen in asymptomatic populations?*
Findings of disc degeneration and bulging discs are commonly seen in the MRIs of asymptomatic individuals. Similarly, a variety of findings occur on the MRIs of knees, shoulders, and hips in an asymptomatic population. One should be careful of interpreting such findings as causative, depending on the other accrued evidence, as described above.

### Provocative Testing:

*Do symptoms shift, vary, resolve or worsen when discussing stressful or emotional topics?*
Watch for changes in symptoms when discussing stressful situations.

*Do symptoms improve with positive affirmations and
challenging triggers or when the patient expresses emotions?*
Ask about changes in symptoms after these therapeutic exercises
are completed.

### Lifetime Review of Symptoms Checklist

Review of Symptoms—Lifetime:

For each of the following, check yes if you have ever had
this symptom or condition and indicate the year it began;
check again if it is still present.

|  | | Yes? | Began When? | Still Present? |
|---|---|---|---|---|
| 1. | Heartburn, acid reflux | ___ | _____ | ___ |
| 2. | Ulcer symptoms or stomach pains | ___ | _____ | ___ |
| 3. | Hiatal hernia | ___ | _____ | ___ |
| 4. | Irritable bowel syndrome | ___ | _____ | ___ |
| 5. | Colitis, spastic colon | ___ | _____ | ___ |
| 6. | Tension headache | ___ | _____ | ___ |
| 7. | Migraine headache | ___ | _____ | ___ |
| 8. | Eczema | ___ | _____ | ___ |
| 9. | Anxiety symptoms and/or panic attacks | ___ | _____ | ___ |
| 10. | Depression | ___ | _____ | ___ |
| 11. | Obsessive-compulsive thought patterns | ___ | _____ | ___ |
| 12. | Eating disorders | ___ | _____ | ___ |
| 13. | Insomnia or trouble sleeping | ___ | _____ | ___ |
| 14. | Fibromyalgia | ___ | _____ | ___ |
| 15. | Back pain | ___ | _____ | ___ |
| 16. | Neck pain | ___ | _____ | ___ |
| 17. | Shoulder pain | ___ | _____ | ___ |

| | Yes? | Began When? | Still Present? |
|---|---|---|---|
| 18. Repetitive stress injury | ____ | _____ | ____ |
| 19. Reflex sympathetic dystrophy (RSD) | ____ | _____ | ____ |
| 20. Temporo-mandibular joint syndrome (TMJ) | ____ | _____ | ____ |
| 21. Chronic tendonitis | ____ | _____ | ____ |
| 22. Carpal tunnel syndrome | ____ | _____ | ____ |
| 23. Numbness, paresthesias | ____ | _____ | ____ |
| 24. Trigeminal neuralgia, facial pain | ____ | _____ | ____ |
| 25. Fatigue or Chronic fatigue syndrome | ____ | _____ | ____ |
| 26. Palpitations | ____ | _____ | ____ |
| 27. Chest pain | ____ | _____ | ____ |
| 28. Hyperventilation | ____ | _____ | ____ |
| 29. Spastic bladder | ____ | _____ | ____ |
| 30. Interstitial cystitis | ____ | _____ | ____ |
| 31. Prostate problems | ____ | _____ | ____ |
| 32. Pelvic pain | ____ | _____ | ____ |
| 33. Muscle tenderness | ____ | _____ | ____ |
| 34. Tachycardia or low blood pressure | ____ | _____ | ____ |
| 35. Tinnitus | ____ | _____ | ____ |
| 36. Dizziness | ____ | _____ | ____ |
| 37. Other symptoms (please list) | ____ | _____ | ____ |

## ACE Questionnaire

1. Did a parent or other adult in the household often or very often… Swear at you, insult you, put you down, or humiliate you? or Act in a way that made you afraid that you might be physically hurt?

2. Did a parent or other adult in the household often or very often… Push, grab, slap, or throw something at you? or Ever hit you so hard that you had marks or were injured?

3. Did an adult or person at least 5 years older than you ever... Touch or fondle you or have you touch their body in a sexual way? or Attempt or actually have oral, anal, or vaginal intercourse with you?

4. Did you often or very often feel that ... No one in your family loved you or thought you were important or special? or Your family didn't look out for each other, feel close to each other, or support each other?

5. Did you often or very often feel that ... You didn't have enough to eat, had to wear dirty clothes, and had no one to protect you? or Your parents were too drunk or high to take care of you or take you to the doctor if you needed it?

6. Was a biological parent ever lost to you through divorce, abandonment, or other reason?

7. Did a parent or other adult in the household often or very often...pushed, grabbed, slapped, or had something thrown at her? or Sometimes, often, or very often kicked, bitten, hit with a fist, or hit with something hard? or Ever repeatedly hit over at least a few minutes or threatened with a gun or knife?

8. Did you live with anyone who was a problem drinker or alcoholic, or who used street drugs?

9. Was a household member depressed or mentally ill, or did a household member attempt suicide?

10. Did a household member go to prison?

### Life Trajectory Interview Description

Review the symptom checklist and place the onset of symptoms in chronological order. Ask permission to search for linkages between onset/exacerbation of symptoms and stressful events.

Ask about symptoms as a child, such as headaches, stomach aches, growing pains, fearfulness, shyness and sensitivity (point out that it is often the "sensitive" people who tend to develop neural pathway pains).

Start with the symptom(s) occurring at the earliest age and ask about what was going on in their life at the time that symptom began. Probe for stressful events and look past medical explanations. "It very well may have been a medical problem, but let's think for a second about what might have been going on in your life at that time."

Proceed with as many of the important symptoms that you can, pointing out linkages as they occur. Provide empathy for them that so many things have happened to them. Point out the pattern of a sensitized danger signal leading to more and more pain and other symptoms over time. Recognize the frustration at not knowing why these are occurring or not getting good pain relief from medications and other interventions. Ask if they are now ready to work on changing the brain in order to reduce or eliminate the pain or other PPD symptoms.

### Personality Traits often linked to PPD

Please check if you would describe yourself as:

1. Having low self-esteem                    _____
2. Being a perfectionist                      _____
3. Having high expectations of yourself       _____
4. Wanting to be good and/or be liked         _____
5. Frequently hostile and/or aggressive       _____
6. Frequently feeling guilt                   _____
7. Feeling dependent on others                _____
8. Being conscientious                        _____
9. Being hard on yourself                     _____
10. Being overly responsible                  _____
11. Often responsible for others              _____
12. Having rage or resentment                 _____

13. Often worrying                                    _____
14. Being sad                                         _____
15. Have difficulty making decisions                  _____
16. A rule-follower                                   _____
17. Have difficulty letting go                        _____
18. Cautious, shy, or reserved                        _____
19. Tend to hold thoughts and feelings in             _____
20. Difficulty standing up for oneself                _____

# References

Aaron LA, Buchwald, D. A review of the evidence for overlap among unexplained clinical conditions. *Annals of Internal Medicine*. 2001, 134: 868-881.

Aaron LA, Bradley LA, Alarcón GS, Alexander RW, Triana-Alexander M, Martin MY, Alberts KR. Psychiatric diagnoses in patients with fibromyalgia are related to health care–seeking behavior rather than to illness. *Arthritis & Rheumatism*. 1996, 39: 436-445.

Abbass A. Somatization: Diagnosing it sooner through emotion-focused interviewing. *Journal of Family Practice*. 2005, 54: 215-24.

Abbass A, Bechard D. Bringing character changes with Intensive Short-term Dynamic Psychotherapy. *Ad Hoc Bulletin of Short-term Dynamic Psychotherapy: Practice and Theory*. 2007, 11: 26-40.

Abbass A, Lovas D, Purdy A. Direct diagnosis and management of emotional factors in chronic headache patients. *Cephalgia*. 2008, 28: 1305-1314.

Abbass A, Kisely S, Kroenke K. Short-term Psychodynamic Psychotherapy for Somatic Symptom Disorders: A systematic review and meta-analysis. *Psychotherapy and Psychosomatics*. 2009, 78: 265–274.

Abbass A, Campbell S, Magee K, Tarzwell R. Intensive short-term dynamic psychotherapy to reduce rates of emergency department return visits for patients with medically unexplained symptoms: preliminary evidence from a pre-post intervention study. *Canadian Journal of Emergency Medicine*. 2009, 11: 529-34.

Abbass A, Campbell S, Hann G, Lenzer I, Tarzwell R. Implementing an emotion-focused consultation service to examine medically unexplained symptoms in the emergency department. *Archives of Medical Psychology.* 2010, 2: 44-52.

Abbass A, Town J, Driessen E. Intensive short-term dynamic psychotherapy: a systematic review and meta-analysis of outcome research. *Harvard Review of Psychiatry.* 2012, 20: 97–108.

Abbass A, Katzman J. The cost-effectiveness of Intensive Short-term Dynamic Psychotherapy. *Psychiatric Annals.* 2013, 43: 496-501.

Abbass A, Kisely S, Rasic D, Town JM, Johansson R. Long-term healthcare cost reduction with intensive short-term dynamic psychotherapy in a tertiary psychiatric service. *Journal of Psychiatric Research.* 2015, 64: 114–20.

Abbass A. *Reaching through resistance: advanced psychotherapy techniques.* Seven Leaves Press, Kansas City. 2015.

Abbass A. The emergence of psychodynamic psychotherapy for treatment resistant patients: Intensive Short-Term Dynamic Psychotherapy. *Psychodynamic Psychiatry.* 2016, 44: 245–80.

Amir M, Kaplan Z, Neumann L, Sharabani R, Shani N, Buskila D. Post-traumatic stress disorder, tenderness and fibromyalgia. *Journal of Psychosomatic Research.* 1997, 42: 607-613.

Anda RF, Felitti VJ, Bremner JD, Walker JD, Whitfield C, Perry BD, Dube SR, Giles WH. The enduring effects of abuse and related adverse experiences in childhood: A convergence of evidence from neurobiology and epidemiology. *European Archives of Psychiatry and Clinical Neuroscience.* 2006, 256: 174-86.

Arkowitz H, Lilienfeld SO. Why science tells us not to rely on eye witness accounts. *Scientific American Mind*. January 1, 2010.

Assor A, Roth G, Deci EL. The Emotional Costs of Parents' Conditional Regard: A Self-Determination Theory Analysis. *Journal of Personality*. 2004, 72: 47-88.

Baliki MN, Petre B, Torbey S, Herrmann KM, Huang L, Schnitzer TJ, Fields HL, Apkarian AV. Corticostriatal functional connectivity predicts transition to chronic back pain. *Nature Neuroscience*. 2012, 15: 1117-1119.

Barsky AJ, Borus JF. Functional somatic syndromes. *Annals of Internal Medicine*. 1999, 130: 910-921.

Barsky AJ, Orav EJ, Bates DW. Somatization increases medical utilization and costs independent of psychiatric and medical comorbidity. *Archives of General Psychiatry*. 2005, 62; 903-10.

Bass, C., Bond, A., Gill, D., & Sharpe, M. Frequent attenders without organic disease in a gastroenterology clinic: Patient characteristics and health care use. *General Hospital Psychiatry*. 1999, 21: 30-38.

Bass C, Peveler R, House A. Somatoform disorders: Severe psychiatric illnesses neglected by psychiatrists. *The British Journal of Psychiatry*. 2001, 179: 11-14.

Beckham JC, Crawford AL, Feldman ME, Kirby AC, Hertzberg MA, Davidson JR, Moore SD. Chronic posttraumatic stress disorder and chronic pain in Vietnam combat veterans. *Journal of Psychosomatic Research*. 1997, 43: 379-389.

Beecher HK. Early care of the seriously wounded man. *Journal of the American Medical Association*. 1951, 145: 193-200.

Bendixen M, Muus KM, Schei B. The impact of child sexual abuse: a study of a random sample of Norwegian students. *Child Abuse & Neglect*. 1994, 18: 837-847.

Bohns VK, Wiltermuth SS. It hurts when I do this (or you do that): Posture and pain tolerance. *Journal of Experimental Social Psychology*. 2012, 48: 341–345.

Boos N, Semmer N, Elfering A, Schade V, Gal I, Zanetti M, Kissling R, Buchegger N, Hodler J, Main CJ. Natural history of individuals with asymptomatic disc abnormalities in magnetic resonance imaging: predictors of low back pain-related medical consultation and work incapacity. *Spine*. 2000, 25: 1484-92.

Borenstein DG, O'Mara JW Jr, Boden SD, Lauerman WC, Jacobson A, Platenberg C, Schellinger D, Wiesel SW. The value of magnetic resonance imaging of the lumbar spine to predict low-back pain in asymptomatic subjects: a seven-year follow-up study. *Journal of Bone and Joint Surgery* (American). 2001, 83-A: 1306-11.

Brinjikji W, Luetmera PH, Comstock B, Breshahan BW, Chenc LE, Deyo RA, Halabig S, Turner JA, Avinsh AL, James K, Wald JT, Kallmes DF, Jarvik JG. Systematic Literature Review of Imaging Features of Spinal Degeneration in Asymptomatic Populations. *American Journal of Neuroradiology*. 2015, 36: 811-816.

Bowlby, J. *A secure base*. Basic Books, New York, 1988.

Brown S, Vaughan C. *Play: How it shapes the brain, opens the imagination, and invigorates the soul*. Penguin Books, New York, 2009.

Burger AJ, Lumley MA, Carty JN, Latsch DV, Thakur ER, Hyde-Nolan ME, Hijazi AM, Schubiner H. A Preliminary Trial of a Novel Psychological Attribution and Emotional Awareness Intervention for Chronic Musculoskeletal Pain. *Journal of Psychosomatic Research*. 2016, 81: 1-8.

Carney DR, Cuddy AJC, Yap AJ. Power Posing: Brief Nonverbal Displays Affect Neuroendocrine Levels and Risk Tolerance. *Psychological Science.* 2010, 21: 1363-1368.

Carragee EJ, Alamin TF, Miller JL, Carragee JM. Discographic, MRI and psychosocial determinants of low back pain disability and remission: a prospective study in subjects with benign persistent back pain. *The Spine Journal.* 2005, 5: 24-35.

Chavooshi B, Mohammadkhani P, Dolatshahi B. A Randomized double-blind controlled trial comparing Davanloo Intensive Short-Term Dynamic Psychotherapy as internet-delivered vs treatment as usual for medically unexplained pain: A 6-Month pilot study. *Psychosomatics.* 2016. 57: 292-300.

Chavooshi B, Mohammadkhani P, Dolatshahi B. Efficacy of Intensive Short-Term Dynamic Psychotherapy for medically unexplained pain: A pilot three-armed randomized controlled trial comparison with mindfulness-based stress reduction. *Psychotherapy and Psychosomatics.* 2016, 85: 123-5.

Cherkin DC, Sherman KJ, Balderson BH, Cook AJ, Anderson ML, Hawkes RJ, Hansen KE, Turner JA. Effect of mindfulness-based stress reduction vs cognitive behavioral therapy or usual care on back pain and functional limitations in adults with chronic low back pain: A randomized clinical trial. *Journal of the American Medical Association.* 2016, 315: 1240-1249.

Christakis NA, Fowler JH. Social contagion theory: examining dynamic social networks and human behavior. *Statistics in Medicine.* 2013, 32: 556-577.

Christensen JO, Knardahl S. Work and back pain: a prospective study of psychological, social and mechanical predictors of back pain severity. *European Journal of Pain.* 2012, 16: 921–933.

Clarke DD. *They can't find anything wrong: 7 keys to understanding, treating, and healing stress.* First Sentient Publications, Boulder, CO. 2007.

Cooper A, Abbass A, Zed J, Bedford L, Sampallia T, Town J. Implementing a psychotherapy service for medically unexplained symptoms in a primary care setting. *Journal of Clinical Medicine.* In press.

Coughlin Della Selva P. Emotional processing in the treatment of psychosomatic disorders. *Journal of Clinical Psychology.* 2006, 62: 539-550.

Creamer P, Hochberg, MC. The relationship between psychosocial variables and pain reporting in osteoarthritis of the knee. *Arthritis and Rheumatism.* 1998, 11: 60-65.

Croskerry P, Abbass A, Wu AW. Emotional Issues in patient safety. *Journal of Patient Safety.* 2010, 6: 199-205.

Crum AJ and Langer EJ. Mindset matters: Exercise and the placebo effect. *Psychological Science.* 2007, 18: 165-171.

Crum AJ, Corbin WR, Brownell KD, Salovey P. Mind over milkshakes: Mindsets, not just nutrients, determine ghrelin response. *Health Psychology.* 2011, 30: 424-429.

Cunningham J, Pearce T, Pearce P. Childhood sexual abuse and medical complaints in adult women. *Journal of Interpersonal Violence.* 1988, 3, 131-144.

Damasio A. *The Feeling of What Happens: Body and Emotion in the Making of Consciousness.* Houghton, Mifflin, Harcourt. New York, 2000.

Davanloo, H. The Technique of Unlocking the Unconscious in Patients Suffering from Functional Disorders. Part I. Restructuring Ego's Defenses, in: *Unlocking the Unconscious.* John Wiley & Sons, Chichester, England, 1990, pp. 283-306.

Davanloo, H. Intensive Short-Term Dynamic Psychotherapy with Highly Resistant Depressed Patients: Part I - Restructuring Ego's Regressive Defenses, in: *Unlocking the Unconscious.* John Wiley & Sons, Chichester, England, 1990, pp. 47-80.

Davanloo H. *Intensive Short-Term Dynamic Psychotherapy.* Wiley Press, Chichester, UK, 2000.

Davanloo, H. Intensive Short-Term Dynamic Psychotherapy, in: Kaplan and Sadock's *Comprehensive Textbook of Psychiatry,* ed. B.J. Sadock & V.A. Sadock. Lippincott, Williams and Wilkins, New York, 2005, pp. 2628-2652.

Deyo RA, Rainville J, Kent DL. What can the history and physical examination tell us about low back pain? *Journal of the American Medical Association.* 1992, 268: 760-765.

Dobie DJ, Kivlahan DR, Maynard C, Bush KR, Davis TM, Bradley KA. Post-traumatic stress disorder in female veterans: Association with self-reported health problems and functional impairment. *Archives of Internal Medicine.* 2004, 164: 394-400.

Drew T, Vo MLH, Wolfe, JM. The invisible gorilla strikes again: Sustained inattentional blindness in expert observers. *Psychological Science.* 2013, 24: 1848-1853.

Eisenberger NI, Jarcho JM, Lieberman MD, Naliboff BD. An experimental study of shared sensitivity to physical pain and social rejection. *PAIN.* 2006, 126: 132 – 138.

Espay AJ, Norris MM, Eliassen JC, Dwivedi A, Smith MS, Banks C, Allendorfer JB, Lang AE, Fleck DE, Linke MJ, Szaflarski JP. Placebo effect of medication cost in Parkinson disease: A randomized double-blind study. *Neurology.* 2015, 84: 794-802.

Falk EB, O'Donnell MB, Cascio CN, Tinney F, Kang Y, Lieberman MD, Taylor SE, An L, Resnicow K, Strecher VJ. Self-affirmation alters the brain's response to health messages and subsequent behavior change. *PNAS (Proceedings of the National Academy of Sciences, USA).* 2015, 112: 1977-1982.

Feldman Barrett L, Simmons WK. Interoceptive predictions in the brain. *Nature Reviews Neuroscience.* 2015, 16: 419-429.

Feldman Barrett, L. *How emotions are made: The secret life of the brain.* Houghton Mifflin Harcourt, Boston, New York, 2017.

Fellitti VJ, Anda RF, Nordenberg D, Williamson DF, Spitz AM, Edwards V, Kross MP, Marks JS. Relationship of childhood abuse and household dysfunction to many of the leading causes of death in adults. The Adverse Childhood Experiences (ACE) study. *American Journal of Preventive Medicine.* 1998, 14: 245-258.

Ferrari R, Russell AS. Effect of a symptom diary on symptom frequency and intensity in healthy subjects. *Journal of Rheumatology.* 2010, 37: 2386-2387.

Ferrari R. Effect of a pain diary use on recovery from acute low back pain (lumbar) sprain. *Rheumatology International.* 2015, 35: 55-59.

Ferrari R, Louw D. Effect of a pain diary use on recovery from acute whiplash injury: a cohort study. *Journal of Zhejiang University, Science B.* 2013, 14: 1049-1053.

Ferreira ML, Zhang Y, Metcalf B, Makovey J, Bennell KL, March L, Hunter DJ. The influence of weather on the risk of pain exacerbation in patients with knee osteoarthritis - a case-crossover study. *Osteoarthritis Cartilage.* 2016, 4: 2042-2047.

Fisher JP, Hassan DT, O'Connor. Minerva. *British Medical Journal*. 1995, 310: 70.

Fonagy P, Allison E The role of mentalizing and epistemic trust in the therapeutic relationship. *Psychotherapy* (Chicago). 2014, 51: 372-80.

Geisser ME, Strader Donnell C, Petzke F, Gracely RH,Clauw DJ, Williams DA. Comorbid somatic symptoms and functional status in patients with fibromyalgia and chronic fatigue syndrome: sensory amplification as a common mechanism. *Psychosomatics*. 2008, 49: 235-42.

Germer C. *The mindful path to self-compassion: Freeing yourself from destructive thoughts and emotions*. The Guilford Press. New York, NY. 2009.

Gillis, ME, Lumley MA, Mosley-Williams A, Leisen JCC, Roehrs T. The health effects of at-home written emotional disclosure in fibromyalgia: A randomized trial. *Annals of Behavioral Medicine*. 2006, 32: 135-146.

Goldberg RT, Pachas WN, Keith D. Relationship between traumatic events in childhood and chronic pain. *Disability and Rehabilitation*. 1999, 21: 23-30.

Goldstein J. *Mindfulness: A Practical Guide to Awakening*. Sounds True, Inc. Boulder, CO. 2013.

Goodwin RD, Hoven CW, Murison R, Hotopf M. Association between childhood physical abuse and gastrointestinal disorders and migraine in adulthood. *American Journal of Public Health*. 2003, 93: 1065-1067.

Gracely RH, Schweinhardt P. Programmed Symptoms: Disparate Effects United by Purpose. *Current Rheumatology Reviews*. 2015, 11, 116-130.

Green CR, Flowe-Valencia H, Rosenblum L, Tait AR. The role of childhood and adulthood abuse among women presenting for chronic pain management. *The Clinical Journal of Pain*. 2001, 17: 359-364.

Grossman P, Tiefenthaler-Gilmer U, Raysz A, Kesper U. Mindfulness training as an intervention for fibromyalgia: evidence of post-intervention and 3-year follow-up benefits in well-being. *Psychotherapy and Psychosomatics*. 2007, 76: 226-233.

Haller H, Cramer H, Lauche R, Dobos, G. Somatoform disorders and medically unexplained symptoms in primary care: a systematic review and meta-analysis of prevalence. *Deutsches Ärzteblatt International*. 2015, 112: 279-287.

Hanscom D. *Back in Control: A spine surgeon's roadmap out of chronic pain*. Vertus Press, Seattle, WA. 2016.

Hashmi JA, Baliki MN, Huang L, Baria AT, Torbey S, Herrmann KM, Schnitzer TJ, Apkarian AV. Shape shifting pain: chronification of back pain shifts brain representation from nociceptive to emotional circuits. *Brain*. 2013, 136: 2751-2768.

Hawkins RD, Abrams TW, Carew TJ, Kandel ER. A cellular mechanism of classical conditioning in Aplysia: activity dependent amplification of presynaptic facilitation. *Science*. 1983, 219: 400-405.

Hebb DO. *The organization of behavior*. New York: Wiley & Sons, 1949.

Henningsen P, Zimmermann T, Sattel H. Medically unexplained physical symptoms, anxiety, and depression: a meta-analytic review. *Psychosomatic Medicine*. 2003, 65: 528-533.

Holmes TH, Rahe RH. The social readjustment rating scale. *Journal of Psychosomatic Research*. 1967, 11: 213-218.

Hsu MC, Schubiner H, Lumley MA, Stracks JS, Clauw DJ, Williams DA. Sustained pain reduction through affective self-awareness in fibromyalgia: a randomized controlled trial. *Journal of General Internal Medicine*. 2010, 25: 1064-70.

Institute of Medicine (US) Committee on Advancing Pain Research, Care, and Education. *Relieving Pain in America: A Blueprint for Transforming Prevention, Care, Education, and Research*. National Academies Press (US), Washington (DC), 2011.

Kabat-Zinn J. *Full catastrophe living*. Random House, NY. 1990.

Kandel ER, Hawkins RD. The biological basis of learning and individuality. *Scientific American*. September 1992, 79-86.

Katon W, Sullivan M, Walker E. Medical symptoms without identified pathology: relationship to psychiatric disorders, childhood and adult trauma, and personality traits. *Annals of Internal Medicine*. 2001, 134: 917-925.

Kirsch I. *The Emperor's New Drugs: Exploding the Antidepressant Myth*. Basic Books, New York. 2010.

Kroenke K. Patients presenting with somatic complaints: epidemiology, psychiatric co-morbidity and management. *International Journal of Methods in Psychiatric Research*. 2003, 12: 34-43.

Kroenke K. The interface between physical and psychological symptoms. *Primary Care Companion to the Journal of Clinical Psychiatry*. 2003, 5: 11-18.

Kroenke K, Rosmalen JG. Symptoms, syndromes, and the value of psychiatric diagnostics in patients who have functional somatic disorders. *Medical Clinics of North America*. 2006, 90: 603-626.

Kroenke K, Spitzer MD, Williams JBW, Lowe B. The Patient Health Questionnaire Somatic, Anxiety, and Depressive Symptom Scales: a systematic review. *General Hospital Psychiatry*. 2010, 32: 345–359.

Kross E, Berman, MG, Mischel W, Smith EE, Wager, TD. Social rejection shares somatosensory representations with physical pain. *Proceedings of the National Academy of Sciences of the USA*. 2011, 108: 6270-6275.

Landa A, Peterson B, Fallon B. Somatoform Pain: A Developmental Theory and Translational Research Review. *Psychosomatic Medicine*. 2012, 74: 717-727.

Latthe P, Mignini L, Gray R, Hills R, Khan K. Factors predisposing women to chronic pelvic pain: systematic review. *British Medical Journal*. 2006, 332: 749-756.

LeDoux J. *The Emotional Brain: The mysterious underpinnings of emotional life*. Touchstone Books, Simon and Schuster, New York, NY. 1996.

Lum TE, Fairbanks RJ, Pennington EC, Zwemet FL. Profiles in patient safety: Misplaced femoral line guidewire and multiple failures to detect the foreign body on chest radiography. *Academic Emergency Medicine*. 2005, 12: 658-662.

Lumley MA, Cohen JL, Borszcz GS, Cano A, Radcliffe AM, Porter LS, Schubiner H, Keefe FJ. Pain and emotion: a biopsychosocial review of recent research. *Journal of Clinical Psychology*. 2011, 67: 942-68.

Lumley MA, Schubiner H, Lockhart NA, Kidwell KM, Harte S, Clauw DJ, Williams DA. Emotional awareness and expression therapy, cognitive-behavioral therapy, and education for fibromyalgia: A cluster-randomized controlled trial. *PAIN*. 2017, 158: 2354-2363.

Luskin F. *Forgive for Good.* HarperCollins, Inc. New York, 2002.

Manu P, Lane TJ, Matthews DA. Somatization disorder in patients with chronic fatigue. *Psychosomatics.* 1989, 30: 388-395.

Mayer EA, Naliboff BD, Chang L, Coutinho SV. Stress and irritable bowel syndrome. *American Journal of Physiology-Gastrointestinal and Liver.* 2001, 280: G519-524.

Martin P. Behavioral management of migraine headache triggers: Learning to cope with triggers. *Current Pain and Headache Reports.* 2010, 14: 221–227.

Meltzer-Brody S, Leserman J, Zolnoun D, Steege J, Green E, Teich A. Trauma and posttraumatic stress disorder in women with chronic pelvic pain. *Obstetrics & Gynecology.* 2007, 109: 902-908.

Merskey, H. Physical and psychological considerations in the classification of fibromyalgia. *The Journal of Rheumatology. Supplement.* 1989, 19: 72-79.

Morgan CA, Hazlett G, Doran A, Garrett S, Hoyt G, Thomas P, Baranoski M, Southwick SM. Accuracy of eyewitness memory for persons encountered during exposure to highly intense stress. *International Journal of Law and Psychiatry.* 2004, 27: 265–279.

Morrison JD. Fatigue as a presenting complaint in family practice. *The Journal of Family Practice.* 1980, 10: 795-801.

Noakes, TD. *Lore of Running.* Oxford University Press Southern Africa. 2001.

Neff K. *Self-compassion: Stop beating yourself up and leave insecurity behind.* HarperCollins Publishers, New York, NY. 2011.

Norman SA, Lumley MA, Dooley JA, Diamond MP. For whom does it work? Moderators of the effects of written emotional disclosure in a randomized trial among women with chronic pelvic pain. *Psychosomatic Medicine.* 2004, 66: 174-183.

Oldfield G. *Chronic Pain: Your key to recovery.* 2QT Limited, UK. 2015.

Pain Recovery Program, TMS/PPD Peer Network, www. tmswiki.org.

Peabody FW. The care of the patient. *Journal of the American Medical Association.* 1927, 88: 877-882.

Pennebaker J. *Writing to Heal: A guided journey to recovering from trauma and emotional upheaval.* New Harbinger Publications, Inc. Oakland, CA. 2004.

Pennebaker J. *Opening Up: The healing power of expressing emotions.* Guilford Press, New York, NY. 1990.

Raphael KG, Chandler HK, Ciccone DS. Is childhood abuse a risk factor for chronic pain in adulthood? *Current Pain and Headache Reports.* 2004, 8: 99-110.

Rief W, Barsky AJ. Psychobiological perspectives on somatoform disorders. *Psychoneuroendocrinology.* 2005, 30: 996-1002.

Raspe H, Hueppe A, Neuhauser H. Back pain, a communicable disease? *International Journal of Epidemiology.* 2008, 37: 69-74.

Russell L, Abbass A, Pohlmann-Eden B, Alder S and Town J. A Preliminary study of reduction in healthcare costs following the application of Intensive Short-Term Dynamic Psychotherapy for psychogenic non-epileptic seizures. *Epilepsy and Behavior.* 2016, 63: 17-19.

Sachs-Ericsson NJ, Sheffler JL, Stanley IH, Piazza JR, Preacher KJ. When emotional pain becomes physical: Adverse childhood experiences, pain, and the role of mood and anxiety disorders. *Journal of Clinical Psychology*. 2017, doi: 10.1002/jclp.22444.

Safran DG, Miller W, Beckman H. Organizational dimensions of relationship-centered care: theory, evidence, and practice. *Journal of General Internal Medicine*. 2006, 21(suppl 1): S9-S15.

Sansone RA, Gaither GA, Sansone LA. Childhood trauma and adult somatic preoccupation by body area among women in an Internal Medicine setting: A pilot study. *International Journal of Psychiatry in Medicine*. 2001, 31: 147-154.

Schechter D. *Think Away your Pain*. Mindbody Medicine Publications, Los Angeles. 2014.

Schechter D, Smith A. Back Pain as a Distraction Pain Syndrome. *Evidence-Based Integrative Medicine*. 2005, 2: 3-8.

Schubiner H, Betzold M. *Unlearn Your Pain* (third edition). Mind Body Publishing, Pleasant Ridge, MI. 2016.

Schubiner H. *Unlearn Your Anxiety and Depression*. Mind Body Publishing, Pleasant Ridge, MI. 2016.

Schulte IE, Petermann F. Familial risk factors for the development ofsomatoform symptoms and disorders in children and adolescents: A systematic review. *Child Psychiatry and Human Development*. 2011, 42: 569–583.

Severeijns RM, Vlaeyen JWS, van den Hout MA, Weber WEJ. Pain catastrophizing predicts pain intensity, disability, and psychological distress independent of the level of physical impairment. *Clinical Journal of Pain*. 2001, 17: 165 – 172.

Sha MC, Callahan CM, Counsell SR, Westmoreland GR, Stump TE, Kroenke K. Physical symptoms as a predictor of health care use and mortality among older adults. *The American Journal of Medicine.* 2005, 118: 301-306.

Sherman JJ, Turk DC, Okifuji A. Prevalence and impact of posttraumatic stress disorder-like symptoms on patients with fibromyalgia syndrome. *Clinical Journal of Pain.* 2000,16: 127-134.

Smyth JM, Stone AA, Hurewitz A. Effects of writing about stressful experiences on symptoms reduction in patients with asthma or rheumatoid arthritis. *Journal of the American Medical Association.* 1999, 281: 1304-1309.

Spertus IL, Yehuda R, Wong CM, Halligan S, Seremetis SV. Childhood emotional abuse and neglect as predictors of psychological and physical symptoms in women presenting to a primary care practice. *Child Abuse & Neglect.* 2003, 27: 1247-1258.

Starfield B, Wray C, Hess K, Gross R, Birk PS, D'Lugoff BC. The influence of patient-practitioner agreement on outcome of care. *American Journal of Public Health.* 1981, 71: 127–131.

Steffens D, Maher CG, Li Q, Ferreira ML, Pereira LSM, Koes BW, Latimer J. Effect of weather on back pain: Results from a case-crossover study. *Arthritis Care and Research.* 2014, 66: 1867-1872.

Stone MJ. The wisdom of Sir William Osler. *American Journal of Cardiology.* 1995, 75: 269 - 276.

Stuart S, Noyes R. Attachment and interpersonal communication in somatization. *Psychosomatics.* 1999, 40: 34-43.

Sumanen M, Rantala A, Sillanmaki LH, Mattila KJ. Childhood adversities experienced by working-age migraine patients. *Journal of Psychosomatic Research.* 2007, 62: 139-143.

Takatalo J, Karppinen J, Niinimäki J, Taimela S, Näyhä S, Järvelin MR, Kyllönen E, Tervonen O. Prevalence of degenerative imaging findings in lumbar magnetic resonance imaging among young adults. *Spine* (Philadelphia). 2009, 34: 1716-21.

Tawakol A, Ishai A, Takx RAP, Figueroa AL, Ali A, Kaiser Y, Truong QA, Solomon CJE, Calcagno C, Mani V, Tang CY, Mulder WJM, Murrough JW, Hoffmann U, Nahrendorf M, Shin LM, Fayad ZA, Pitman RK. Relation between resting amygdalar activity and cardiovascular events: a longitudinal and cohort study. *The Lancet*. 2017, 389: 834-845.

Thompson WG, Longstreth G, Drossman D, Heaton K, Irvine E, Müller-Lissner S. Functional bowel disorders and functional abdominal pain. *Gut*. 1999, 45: II43-II47.

Tietjen GE, Peterlin BL. Childhood abuse and migraine: epidemiology, sex differences, and potential mechanisms. *Headache*. 2011, 51: 869-879.

Town JM, Driessen E. Emerging evidence for intensive short-term dynamic psychotherapy with personality disorders and somatic disorders. *Psychiatric Annals*. 2013, 43: 502–507.

van Dessel N, den Boeft M, van der Wouden JC, Kleinstäuber M, Leone SS, Terluin B, Numans ME, van der Horst HE, van Marwijk H. Non-pharmacological interventions for somatoform disorders and medically unexplained physical symptoms (MUPS) in adults. *Cochrane Database of Systematic Reviews*. 2014, 11: CD011142.

van Houdenhove B, Neerinckx E, Lysens R, Vertommen H, van Houdenhove L, Onghena P, et. al. Victimization in chronic fatigue and fibromyalgia in tertiary care: A controlled study on prevalence and characteristics. *Psychosomatics*. 2001, 42: 21-28.

Vissers RJ, Kalbfleisch N. The Difficult Patient. In Rosen's *Emergency Medicine: Concepts and Clinical Practice*, 8th edition. Saunders, NY, 2013.

Wessely S, Nimnuan C, SharpeM. Functional somatic syndromes: one or many? *The Lancet*. 1999, 354: 936-939.

Whitehead WE, Bosmajian L, Zonderman A, Costa P, Schuster M. Symptoms of psychologic distress associated with irritable bowel syndrome. *Gastroenterology*. 1988, 95: 709-714.

Whittemore JW. Paving the royal road: An overview of conceptual and technical features in the graded format of Davanloo's Intensive Short-term Dynamic Psychotherapy. *International Journal of Intensive Short-term Dynamic Psychotherapy*. 1996, 11: 21 39.

Yunus MB. Fibromyalgia and overlapping disorders: the unifying concept of central sensitivity syndromes. *Seminars in Arthritis and Rheumatism*. 2007, 36: 339-5.

# Resources

## Available Online:

PPD/TMS Peer Network: Peer-run support website with information, interviews, an online recovery program, and a list of practitioners: www.tmswiki.org

Allan Abbass, MD: publications and courses: www.allanabbass.com

Courses in ISTDP: istdpinstitute.com/

Howard Schubiner, MD: www.unlearnyourpain.com

Pain Psychology Center: Counseling center specializing in PPD therapy via phone and Skype: www.painpsychologycenter.com

David Hanscom, MD: www.backincontrol.com

Stress Illness Recovery Practitioners Association: www.sirpauk.com

Psychophysiologic Disorders Association: www.ppdassociation.org

## Books to Educate Patients About Psychophysiologic Disorders:

Anderson, Frances and Sherman, Eric. *Pathways to Pain Relief.* 2013.

Clarke, David. *They Can't Find Anything Wrong.* 2007.

Hanscom, David. *Back in Control.* 2016.

Oldfield, Georgie. *Chronic Pain: Your Key to Recovery.* 2014.

Ozanich, Steven. *The Great Pain Deception.* 2012.

Sachs, Nicole. *The Meaning of Truth.* 2013.

 Sarno, John. *Healing Back Pain, The Divided Mind, The Mindbody Prescription, Mind Over Back Pain.* 1982-2006.

Schechter, David. *Think Away Your Pain.* 2014.

Schubiner, Howard. *Unlearn Your Pain, Unlearn Your Anxiety and Depression.* Both 2016.

Selfridge, Nancy. *Freedom from Fibromyalgia.* 2001.

Siegel, Ronald; Urdang, Michael; Johnson, Douglas. *Back Sense.* 2001.

## Books for Professionals on ISTDP:

Abbass AA. *Reaching through resistance: advanced psychotherapy techniques.* Seven Leaves Press, Kansas City. 2015.

Coughlin P. *Maximizing Effectiveness in Dynamic Psychotherapy.* Routledge, Abingdon, UK. 2016.

Davanloo H. *Intensive Short-Term Dynamic Psychotherapy.* Wiley Press, Chichester, UK. 2000.

Frederickson J. *Co-Creating Change: Effective Dynamic Therapy Techniques.* Seven Leaves Press, Kansas City. 2013.

# Index

# About the Authors

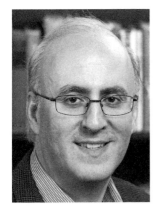

ALLAN ABBASS, MD, is a psychiatrist and professor and founding director of the Centre for Emotions and Health at Dalhousie University in Halifax, Canada. He studied psychosomatic based therapy at McGill University with Dr. Habib Davanloo. In 2002, he founded The Centre for Emotions and Health for the study of psychosomatic medicine. Dr. Abbass has won departmental, regional, and national awards for excellence in education.

His innovative program to diagnose and treat emotional contributors to medically unexplained symptoms in the emergency department won a Quality Award and a national designation as a "Canadian Leading Practice." He has been consulted widely by governments, universities, and health agencies and has provided over 250 invited presentations around the world. He provides ongoing video-recording-based psychotherapy training to professionals in several countries around the world.

In addition, Dr. Abbass has been awarded seventeen research grants and has over 200 publications. His first book *Reaching through Resistance* is widely viewed as a landmark volume on current accelerated dynamic therapy methods.

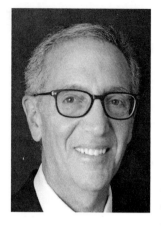

HOWARD SCHUBINER, MD is a specialist in internal medicine and is the director of the Mind Body Medicine Program at Providence Hospital in Southfield, Michigan. He is a Clinical Professor at the Michigan State University College of Human Medicine. He has conducted research resulting in more than 100 publications and has given more than 250 professional lectures nationally and internationally. Dr. Schubiner is on the board of directors of the Psychophysiologic Disorders Association and is a senior teacher of mindfulness meditation. He has been included on the list of the Best Doctors in America since 2003. His other books include *Unlearn Your Pain* and *Unlearn Your Anxiety and Depression*. Dr. Schubiner lives in the Detroit area with his wife of thirty-four years and has two adult children.